BN

FOOD FOR HEALTH, FOOD FOR WEALTH

THE ANTHROPOLOGY OF FOOD AND NUTRITION

General editor: *Helen Macbeth*

Volume 1
Food and the Status Quest. An Interdisciplinary Perspective
Edited by *Polly Wiessner* and *Wulf Schiefenhovel*

Volume 2
Food Preferences and Taste: Continuity and Change
Edited by *Helen Macbeth*

Volume 3
Food for Health, Food for Wealth: The Performance of Ethnic and Gender Identities by Iranian Settlers in Britain
By *Lynn Harbottle*

FOOD FOR HEALTH, FOOD FOR WEALTH

*The Performance of Ethnic and Gender
Identities by Iranian Settlers in Britain*

Lynn Harbottle

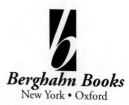

Berghahn Books
New York • Oxford

First published in 2000 by **Berghahn Books**

www.berghahnbooks.com

Library of Congress Cataloging-in-Publication Data

Harbottle, Lynn.
   Food for health, food for wealth : the performance of ethnic and
gender identities by Iranian settlers in Britain / Lynn Harbottle.
      p. cm. -- (The anthropology of food and nutrition ; v.3)
   Includes bibliographical references and index.
   ISBN 1-57181-740-9 (alk. paper)
   1. Iranians--Food--Great Britain. 2. Iranians--Great Britain--
Social life and customs. 3. Women innigrants--Great Britain--
Social conditions. 4. Women--Iran--Social conditions. 5. Food
habits--Great Britain. 6. Food habits--Iran. I. Title. II.
Series.
      DA125.I68 H37 2000
      394.1'08991'55041--dc21
                                                    98-045425
                                                         CIP

British Library Cataloguing-in-Publication Data
A catalogue record for this book is available from the British Library.

Printed in the UK on acid-free paper.

ISBN 1-57181-740-9

To Maureen Duggan – with thanks for introducing me to research and for lending me the book *Daughter of Persia*, which ultimately led to this study.

CONTENTS

FIGURES

ACKNOWLEDGEMENTS

Primarily, I wish to thank all the Iranian individuals and families who collaborated in the undertaking of this study. I am also particularly grateful to Ronnie Frankenberg, Judith Monks, Soraya Tremayne, Fatimeh Rabiee, Iraj Hoshi, Azam Torab, Shirene Pezeshgi, Pnina Werbner and Anne Murcott for their advice and encouragement at various stages of the writing process.

1. INTRODUCTION

The origins of this study date back to the Iranian revolution of 1979. At that time I was an undergraduate student in Manchester and had become friendly with a group of Iranian students there. I observed the immediate impact of the Islamic revolution upon their lives, and, over subsequent years, I also noted how British perceptions of Iranians were transformed as a result of international media coverage of those events. Previously, as western allies, Iranians were often portrayed to be progressive, wealthy and intelligent, but, in the wake of the revolution, it seemed to me that they were redefined. Suddenly, Iran was perceived once more to be a third world nation, and its people were now thought to be illiterate peasants and religious fundamentalists (Dorman, 1979).

For me, the media image of black-shrouded women, carrying red roses to mourn the loss of their loved ones, became one of the most potent and deeply moving symbols of the revolution. Ironically, this image also appears to have resulted in powerful and long-lasting stereotypes, within Britain and other western nations, regarding the oppressed status of Iranian women (Hoodfar, 1993). Over the ensuing years, I became increasingly intrigued by the disjunction between these stereotypes and the assertiveness actually demonstrated by the Iranian women I knew. Moreover, as a nutritionist I was also fascinated by the considerable respect these women derived from their domestic food-work. Their apparently high status contrasted with the position of dietitians within the N.H.S., who continually struggled to distance themselves from the food connotations of their work and so to attain 'scientific credibility'.

Originally, the study upon which this book is based was designed to combine nutritional and anthropological methods. However, during the research process both my identity as a nutritionist and the shape of this project were to undergo further transformations (as detailed in the Appendix). Ultimately then, this book is concerned, not with a nutrition survey, as I had originally intended, but with an exploration of the significance of particular food preparation and eating practices in the performance of ethnic and gender identities by Iranian settlers in Britain. Ethnographic fieldwork was carried out over a two and a half year period and comprised interviews and participant observations with Iranian men, women and children in northern Britain (further details of the research procedure are given in the Appendix). Even at a preliminary stage I noticed that conversations about food almost inevitably seemed to result in discussions of identity. For example, in response to a question about the nutritional rationale for selecting shoulder of lamb, a forty minute debate between one interviewee, Asli, and her husband, Mahmood, ensued in which they considered the impact of western influences, first upon the diet in Iran, and then upon their cultural identities (excerpts from this interview are included in Chapters 4 and 6).

Food, Identity and Performance

The study of identity has become a major focus within contemporary social and cultural theory (Moore, 1994: 2), and within anthropological and sociological research into food and eating (Caplan, 1997: 9; Warde, 1997:197). The term identity is derived from the Latin root *identitas* or 'the same', and the notion simultaneously invokes both relations of similarity on the one hand, and of difference on the other (Jenkins, 1996: 3). Identity is a crucial matter in human social interaction, involving as it does the establishment and signification of relationships of sameness and of difference between individuals and groups. Accordingly we define and understand who we are, and who others are in relation to us.

As Jenkins observes (1996: 4) the verb 'to identify' is an integral aspect of identity-formation, i.e. 'identity is not "just there", it must always be established' in the flux of social interaction. This process begins at birth and continues throughout the life-cycle. Identity is not then an intrinsic property of an individual, or an essential attribute which is simply given meaning within a particular sociocultural environment, but, rather, identity exists only in a social context. Nevertheless, individuals often perceive certain identities to be based upon, or to be naturally derived from innate features, such as sex characteristics. However, even the biological significations attributed to bodily features such as 'male' and 'female' genitalia are themselves socially determined. Those identities which are established early in childhood, and which include gender and ethnic identities, are most commonly perceived to be essential and pervasive. These primary identities also tend to hold the greatest potency in later life and may be less malleable than other, later-established identities, such as those associated with occupation and peer group, although this is not always the case (Jenkins, 1996: 62).

The notion of social identity incorporates not only internal referents, i.e. how we see and present ourselves, but also encompasses external definition, that is how we are perceived and categorised by others, and as I suggested earlier in relation to British Iranians, there may be considerable disjunction between the two. Thus identification should be conceptualised as an ongoing process involving the dialectic interplay of both internal and external referents. During this study, I began to realise that for Iranian settlers in Britain the task of preserving their ethnic identities, while functioning in a society which was perceived by them to be hostile and discriminatory, was of great importance and moreover seemed to involve a considerable amount of work. I also began to understand that food provided an important medium for the maintenance of ethnic identity and it gradually became clear to me that through their diverse food preparation and consumption practices, men, women and children engaged in variable performances of their ethnic identities, according to their positions within the wider society and the varying significance of internal and external processes of identification.

At an early stage in the field work, I began to feel that Claude Fischler's notion of incorporation held particular resonance with these data. Food, as Fischler has attested (1988), carries a powerful symbolic potential and is therefore very important to identity-formation, at both an individual and at a collective level. His notion of 'incorporation' recognises the symbolic aspects of ingestion by which the culturally ascribed properties of a food are assimilated by the embodied social person, together with the nutrients which are absorbed and integrated within the cells and tissues. As a nutritionist-turned-anthropologist, Fischler's theory appealed to me, as I felt that it effectively bridged the gap between anthropological meaning-centred concerns and the nutritional preoccupation with the corporeality of the human body. Moreover, it seemed to accord with the accounts of Iranian women who, in undertaking their domestic food-provisioning tasks, were not only expressly concerned to maintain the ethnic identities of their families but who also gave commensurate attention to ensuring the nutritional and aesthetic acceptability of the food they served. Thus as one participant, Goli, observed, the food she prepared must be 'delicious and nutritious' and must be 'satisfying' to her family.

In addition to the explicit concerns of the participants regarding ethnic and national identity, my own background and observations had led me to a preoccupation with the subject of gender identities and status, as these are articulated through the medium of food, and in particular food-work. Thus, a further set of research questions was generated in relation to the dissonance between western stereotypes regarding the position of Muslim women and the actual status and respect they apparently attained through the performance of their domestic food-work. The fieldwork also highlighted the ways in which Iranian women employed food and food-work as a means by which to attest the superiority of their own female identities in relation to those of British women (and over women from different regions in Iran). Although domestic food-work provided a key medium for the performance and enhancement of female identity, it became apparent that food-work within the public sphere did not offer the same opportunities to Iranian men, rather their gender identities may have been subtly undermined by engaging in this relatively unskilled sector.

With regard to the assertion of male identities, it has been suggested that in many societies an avoidance of female-associated roles and activities, including cooking, is necessary to the effective performance of masculinity (Fürst, 1991: 120). In this study, the significant involvement of Iranian men in food-provisioning, both within the domestic arena and within the fast-food trade, in relatively unskilled work generally associated with women and other migrants, led me to consider how these activities might shape and modify their identities as men.

The data suggest that a considerable degree of flexibility was permitted in both men's and women's performances of gender, and this plasticity seemed to be attributable to the fundamental significance ascribed to sex differences in the determination of Iranian gender identities. Gender identities are formed partially through the cultural interpretation of bodily features (including male and female genitalia) and partly through performance, or social enactment. The relative weighting of these two elements in the construction of identities is, as Moore has observed, cross-culturally variable (1994: 38–39). The findings from this study are of particular interest because it has been supposed that gender identities are more likely to be flexible and fluid in societies where greater significance is ascribed to behavioural aspects (Moore, 1994: 40). Moore also observes that where greater import is given to bodily attributes, identities may often be perceived to be essential, pervasive and unchanging, yet in this study it becomes apparent that it is precisely because the categories of male and female are thought to be sharply defined by their associated sexual characteristics, that Iranian men and women enjoy considerable latitude in their performances of gender roles, such that, for example, men are able to undertake everyday domestic meal preparation without affecting their status as men. However, although behaviour may not be considered to alter what is perceived to be the essential nature of men and women, it may result in their categorisation as more or less valued or ideal role models.

In this context performance is understood, not in the restricted context of formal ritual (although it also incorporates these moments) but in the more mundane sense – as integral to the flow of social life. Performance encompasses a series of culturally appropriate activities or roles, through which actors strike a balance between the constraints of the role and the idiosyncrasies of their own individual biographies (Frankenberg, 1986). Each actor plays a role in a specific way and his/her performance will be interpreted variably by different observers. In the process, new insights may be derived and new symbols may be generated which may be incorporated within subsequent performances (Turner, 1982: 79). Accordingly, everyday activities, including eating behaviour and food provisioning, offer the opportunity for the protagonists involved to enact (and to modify) a number of diverse identities, including those of ethnicity and gender. For example, in their cooking of *ghormeh-sabzi* Iranian women draw upon past and present aesthetic and nutritional knowledge, as well as their individual culinary skills, as they perform the tasks of washing, chopping, cooking, garnishing and serving the meal. These processes and the resulting product serve to mark their particular regional identities and to reinforce their national identities as Iranian, while at the same time incorporating change (as is discussed in Chapter 4).

Eating behaviour, and commensality, is an important means by which cultural and other identities are established and enacted, and as these findings suggest, may provide a particularly potent means of asserting ethnic identity for migrants, such as these Iranian settlers, and of marking their difference from the majority population. The consumption of some foods and avoidance of others, as well as the decisions made regarding who we eat with, how much we consume and the appropriate etiquette for the occasion, facilitate culturally sanctioned performances through which we relay crucial information about who we are. As Fischler has argued (1988) the principle of incorporation is important in terms of both the individual and collective aspects of identity-formation. Thus, not only does the eater incorporate the symbolic properties of the food consumed, but, at the same time, the absorption of that food serves to integrate the consumer within a particular food culture.

In this study, Iranian children demonstrate particular flexibility and variety in their food consumption practices, for example, eating food from a variety of ethnic cuisines, as well as Iranian dishes and consuming home cooked meals and takeaways, as well as dining out occasionally. Accordingly, we may infer that such performances demonstrate the complexity and multivocality of their ethnic identities. However, the apparently playful approach with which these young people engage in food consumption also raises a further question regarding the actual significance of food and eating in relation to processes of identity-construction. Although Fischler's work implies that food consumption is always a significant business in terms of its identity implications, and Iranian women certainly seem to undertake their food-provisioning tasks from this perspective, Warde (1997: 203) suggests that this may not always be so. Rather, he argues that this kind of play may actually represent relatively superficial aspects of individual identity-formation. He contends that although these signifiers (associated with style and status) have comprised the main focus of recent consumption studies, they may be of only transient importance (Warde, 1997: 203). Long-term identity-formation, Warde asserts, may be more profoundly influenced by deeper-rooted processes which invoke emotional security and a sense of social belonging. In this study, the kind of work that Iranian women engage in, to ensure the regular (although not necessarily daily) consumption of Iranian cooked meals, involves an investment of time, energy and love. The food produced in this way appears to carry an affective potency that commercially prepared food and other meals consumed outside the home seem generally to lack. In this case the consumption of the family meal within the home, through the mediation of these affective bonds, is probably of greater lasting significance in processes of individual and collective identity-construction.

It is not only through food consumption that identities may be articulated and transformed. The practices involved in food production also constitute important means by which identities, in particular gender roles, are performed. For example, this study illustrates how, by engaging in a series of culturally regulated activities essential to the preparation of a family meal or even of a single food, such as rice (as described in Chapter 6), Iranian women in Britain not only demonstrate their prowess as cooks, but in the process, they also convey information about their values and they reinforce their identities as women, wives and mothers. On other occasions, for example the preparation of commercially produced takeaway food by Iranian men, the specific performances engaged in may serve to disguise, rather than to reinforce, cultural identities and to undermine, rather than to enhance gender identities.

Clearly, and as the preceding account has demonstrated, there is no simple relationship between food, performance and processes of identity-construction. Rather, the relationship, like the concept of identity itself, seems to be complex, shifting and context-dependent. Moreover, as I have suggested, the symbolic potency of food may itself be highly variable, such that food practices may be of relatively minor significance in relation to identity-formation within the ethnic majority. However, for minority groups, such as these Iranian settlers, for whom identity-construction may be a more conscious and potentially a more problematic process, food consumption may be ascribed much greater symbolic weight.

Ultimately, these data contribute to a contemporary body of British anthropological and sociological research into food and eating which has evolved from the pioneering work of the structuralist school in the sixties and seventies. In particular, the contributions of Claude Lévi-Strauss and Mary Douglas, in their recognition of the significance of food as a cultural system, have been very influential. Lévi-Strauss demonstrated that food is 'good to think' with and that by deciphering the codes applied to food and eating practices we can achieve greater understanding of the structure of thought of the people under study (1968: 87). The work of Mary Douglas (for example, 1970; 1982) shows how food and eating may symbolise the social order of specific groups and that culture mediates not only what counts as food but also how we eat it.

Although the search for symbolic meaning has remained central to current anthropological research on food, this study illustrates that it provides only a partial understanding of the complex nature of food consumption practices. Early structuralist analyses were rightly criticised by materialists who argued for the need to apply a historical perspective (e.g. Mennell, 1985), to take into consideration political economic forces (e.g. Mintz, 1985) and nutritional and ecological influences (Harris, 1986). Moreover, the intellectualist approach of the structuralists, which implies the existence of static and unchanging social systems, overlooks the transformative capacity of the social order, the importance of individual agency and the considerable plasticity in people's behaviour within a system. An analytical approach which incorporates a focus on performance provides a behavioural perspective which complements the rigid structuralist approach.

This book illustrates how a multifaceted analysis is required in order to comprehend how specific food consumption practices and ideologies evolve and develop. For example, participants in this study clearly articulated how they perceived food to be important in maintaining bodily health, and how this consideration was vital to them in making their food consumption choices. It also became apparent that their understandings of the relative health properties of Iranian and British foodstuffs had been influenced by the long-term political manoeuvrings of British governments in Iranian affairs. Furthermore, the structural position of Iranians as migrants, living in a society they considered to be discriminatory, is shown to be an important factor affecting their occupational choices and the type of food served in Iranian-owned takeaway outlets. Whereas a purely symbolic approach would have offered only a partial understanding of the food consumption practices of this group, by integrating political-economic perspectives with an awareness of these Iranian settlers as embodied subjects, engaging in a range of performative roles, I aim to achieve a more holistic and complex analysis of the significance of food and feeding work within this ethnic minority group.

Iranian Migrants in Britain

This study population is comprised of Shi'ite Iranians, predominantly from middle class backgrounds. The majority are permanent residents in Britain but the sample also includes a small number of temporary residents (all postgraduate students). The Iranian population in Britain has been estimated at around 28,000, according to data from the last (1991) census (Thurman, personal communication, O.P.C.S., 1993). These statistics, which are based on place of birth and therefore exclude all those born in Britain of Iranian parents, are considered to be a gross underestimate. The population is centred mainly around London, Brighton and Greater Manchester, with smaller clusters forming around other cities, including Birmingham, Leeds, Sheffield and Newcastle-upon-Tyne. Iranians are extremely heterogeneous in terms of ethnic, religious and political affiliations, with a high degree of social fragmentation. They comprise, for example, Armenians, Assyrians, Kurds and Turkmans, Jews, Bahais, Zorastrians and Christians. This study focuses on only one religious group – Shi'ites – but from a variety of regional and ethnic backgrounds.

Prior to the Islamic revolution of 1979, there was a relatively constant flow of fairly affluent Iranian students, many returning to Iran upon the completion of their studies. In the aftermath of the revolution, and the Iran-Iraq war, increasing numbers of migrants and refugees (more diverse in social class, religious and ethnic backgrounds) arrived in Europe and North America, commonly seeking permanent residence (Gilanshah, 1990; Kamalkhani, 1991; Bagheri, 1992; Lipson, 1992). There has been extensive socio-political documentation of the causes and consequences of the fall of the Shah and of the revolution in Iran (see for example Ramzani, 1986; Fuller, 1991; Zonis, 1991). It is not within the scope of this account to reiterate such theories. From an anthropological perspective, Fischer (1980) and Fischer and Abedi (1990) have undertaken detailed analysis of the historical, political, religious and cultural background to the revolution and of the ongoing influence of Islam in the everyday lives of the Iranian people.

Other anthropological studies set in Iran have tended to focus on the position and spiritual roles of Iranian Shi'ite women (for example, Beck and Keddie, 1979; Jamzadeh and Mills, 1986; Afshah, 1993; Torab, 1996), whilst medical anthropologists such as Good (1977) have explored the psycho-social and cultural dimensions and, in particular, the semantics of illness in this society.

Migration: Cultural Dislocation or Transformation?

The rapid exodus of migrants from Iran to the west, which was precipitated by the Islamic revolution has resulted in considerable interest in their welfare and cultural adaptation, particularly among social science and health researchers in North America and Scandinavia (for example, Kamalkhani, 1988: 152–59; Bagheri, 1992; Fathi, 1991; Lipson, 1992). To date, there appears to have been no comparable research based in Britain.

Migration is generally considered to be a very stressful experience, often accompanied by rapid and dislocating cultural changes (Bagheri, 1992; Clinton-Davis and Fassil, 1992; Lipson, 1992). The exposure of migrants to a new culture, with divergent belief systems, political structures and values, and in which social and individual identities are constructed and performed in distinct or unfamiliar ways may give rise to considerable sociocultural dissonance and to problems of identity. Some psychological and psychiatric studies suggest that Iranians may encounter more profound emotional difficulties and maladjustment than other groups of settlers (Bagheri, 1992; Lipson, 1992). Anthropological analyses also indicate a particularly high degree of discordance and social alienation among Iranians who have settled in western societies (Pliskin, 1987: 106–32; Kamalkhani, 1988: 152–59; 1991). Those who are isolated, have language difficulties or experience a decline in their socioeconomic status may also suffer a loss of self-esteem which may exacerbate problems of identity. It has also been suggested that involuntary refugees (particularly if subjected to physical or psychological trauma) may encounter greater difficulties in settling in a foreign environment than do intentional migrants (Bagheri, 1992).

The positive aspects of intercultural adaptation and identity-formation have been largely obscured by a preoccupation among researchers with cultural difficulties and conflict, and such research is often based on the premise that assimilation is desirable (Harbottle, 1995: 20–25). In a number of these studies somewhat essentialist notions of culture are inferred, in which migrants are often perceived to be caught between two oppositionally situated and static cultures. However, as I have already observed, Iranian culture is polyvocal and complex, comprising numerous internal ethnic, religious, linguistic and political groups and having been exposed to sustained and powerful western influences, as well as to considerable social and cultural disruptions since the Islamic revolution.

The process of migration, whatever the motivating forces involved, leads to the exposure of individuals to new cultural systems (and cuisines). Although for some the crossing of cultural and geographical boundaries may result in identity-conflict and the kinds of problems detailed above, for many others the experience allows for positive identity fusions and transformations (Fischer and Abedi, 1990: 255; Gardner, 1995: vii), as the data from this study illustrate (see also Harbottle, 1995). Fischer and Abedi's view of migrants, which considers them to belong to two social systems which are dynamically intertwined, exemplifies a recent trend within postmodern anthropology, away from the representation of cultures as integrated and bounded wholes, towards analyses which emphasise difference, diversity and contestation and which recognise culture to comprise a multiplicity of signifying practices.

Nevertheless, within the collective imagination of a group, notions of stable communities and 'pure' identities remain highly significant, particularly in situations of perceived threat (Werbner, 1997: 3–4). For migrants exposed to strange and sometimes hostile social environments, the maintenance of a sense of cultural cohesion and stability may therefore be much more important than for the ethnic majority. Kalka (1988) has observed that the continuance of traditional food habits may be one important means of preserving a sense of cultural identity, and other aspects of cultural production, such as language and music, may also acquire increased significance in this context. This study considers the relationship between the tendencies towards 'tradition' and continuity on the one hand and innovation on the other, and, for example, explores how mothers, through the performance of their domestic food-preparation tasks, work to maintain a sense of cultural and culinary stability. Simultaneously, they also incorporate minor modifications during these performances, and engage in subtle transformations of their own identities and those of their families.

The Structure of this Book

The different roles and structural positions of men, women, and indeed children, apparently delimit or facilitate their performances of cultural and gender identities in variable ways. The following chapters explore the significance of food-provisioning and consumption in relation to the performance of those identities. First, however, a more detailed review of some of the key anthropological and other social science contributions to the study of food and eating is given in Chapter 2. Anthropological perspectives are concerned with the ways in which eating practices are elaborated according to cultural mores. For example, they examine the reasons why, cross-culturally, only a limited selection of all that is theoretically edible is actually consumed as food and how, from infancy, individuals learn the deep-rooted culturally defined rules regarding 'what is to count as food and which foods are appropriate for what occasions...' (Murcott, 1988). The relevance of these anthropological (and sociological) approaches is considered in relation to contemporary anthropological research and to the data from this study. Taking sugar as an example, Chapter 3 demonstrates that although the taste for this substance is recognised to be based on an innate predisposition, it is nevertheless socio-culturally mediated in very particular ways. In the case of Shi'ite Iranians in Britain, the research findings illustrate how the intersection of health beliefs and political and economic forces result in distinctive symbolic valuations of this substance.

As I mentioned at the outset, this research was initially designed from a nutritional perspective. However, this changed as my own identity shifted and as I responded to the data emerging from the early stages of fieldwork. The nutrition approach tends to view food in terms of its nutrient composition and effects upon the body's metabolic processes. If dietary beliefs and food habits are observed by nutritionists, it is usually with the intent of facilitating dietary change. To date, there has been limited diffusion of knowledge between the fields of nutrition and anthropology, although Tan and Wheeler's (1983) study of the hot-cold beliefs of Chinese mothers in London and Kalka's work on the changing diets of Gujaratis in

Britain, which suggests that the maintenance of traditional food habits may be important in preserving a sense of stability and cohesion (1988), are notable exceptions. However, recently, 'the Nation's Diet' research programme, directed by Anne Murcott, has resulted in a greater measure of interdisciplinary exchange, as evidenced by Caplan's recent volume 'Food, Health and Identity' (1997). This addresses issues of concern to both fields (for example, the response of the public to receiving dietary advice, the sustained significance of the family meal and the subject of vegetarianism), and of more specific relevance to this text, Bradby's medical sociological study of the health beliefs and food practices of Punjabi women in Glasgow. This text contributes to the cross-disciplinary dialogue now emerging.

Having outlined the key approaches taken to the study of food and eating, the focus then shifts more fully to the empirical data arising from this study. In Chapters 4 and 5 the domestic food-work of Iranian women is examined, illustrating how their understandings of health interweave consideration of the nutritional and aesthetic aspects of food preparation with attention to the symbolic aspects of consumption and identity. As previously stated both Iranian culture and cuisine are polyvocal and these chapters demonstrate how national, regional, global and local cultural influences and identities are performed and contested through variations and modifications in meal preparation. The task of maintaining the health and integrity of the family through appropriate food production is a major responsibility for these women and through enacting this role they apparently derive considerable respect and status within the community.

Although food consumption may be assumed to be a pleasurable experience, pursued with the intent of meeting needs and satisfying desires, because food physically passes through body boundaries it may also be a dangerous activity (Fischler, 1988). Hence, the act of incorporation may be associated with ambivalence and anxiety, linked, for example, with biological risks such as poisoning, or with fears regarding symbolic pollution. Chapter 6 develops Fischler's theory by considering the dilemma of Iranian women obliged to buy foodstuffs which have undergone a series of (market-based) production processes, which are perceived to have changed the substance of the food in deleterious ways. It appears from these data that the anxieties of Iranian women regarding the ingestion of food containing toxins may at a deeper level also represent a fear of contamination by western cultural values.

Adapting Lévi-Strauss's culinary triangle (1966), the chapter further analyses how Iranian women are able positively to transform potentially dangerous raw ingredients into nourishing and satisfying cooked meals. This is achieved through their daily food preparation rituals, the investment of skill and the application of specific cooking techniques and ingredients (often grown in known and trusted environments, for example by their families in Iran). In the process they are also able to maintain a sense of culinary coherence and continuity.

If women are responsible for maintaining and reinforcing the identities of themselves and their families as Iranian, their male partners apparently work to disguise and thereby to protect their identities. Chapter 7 explores why a considerable number of Iranian men (and a small number of women) seek employment in the fast-food business. In this chapter, the complex sociocultural and political-economic forces influencing the occupational choices of these often well-educated individuals, and the resultant emergence of an ethnic enclave economy are considered. The participation of these men in a relatively unskilled occupation, together with the respect accorded to their partners for their domestic food responsibilities, subverts any simplistic notions of a clear association between public/private: male/female and high/low status and reveals how migration may create new opportunities for the negotiation of gender and familial power relations.

The chapter also considers why, although Iranian-owned takeaways abound, few sell identifiably Iranian foods. Chapter 8 continues this theme, to examine why, despite the sophistication of this cuisine, there are few successful Iranian restaurants in Britain. The apparent despoiling of Iranian identity wrought by international responses to the Islamic revolution of 1979 is shown to be a major factor resulting in the failure of Iranian restaurant owners to enlist the interests of British customers. The prevailing negative stereotypes of Iran and Iranians have seemingly undermined any interest in their cuisine or other aspects of their culture by the ethnic majority and the performative response in the face of perceived threat appears to be dissimulation and other defensive strategies. Processes of *self*-stigmatisation and the desire to avoid further rejection by the majority population, as well as internal divisions and fragmentation within the Iranian settler population have also apparently contributed to a reticence among Iranian entrepreneurs to engage in the commercial production of Iranian food.

Chapters 9 and 10 examine more closely the assertion of gender identities through the medium of food, for example, how individual foods carry specific gender connotations, and the gendering of food-preparation tasks. Food is not only a source of sustenance, it is also an economic commodity and the relative weighting of economic, aesthetic and affective values may have considerable bearing on the status derived from food-work. Whereas women's domestic cooking performances involve the investment of a considerable amount of emotional energy, as well as time and skill, which will be incorporated by the family along with the food consumed, their partners' food-work within the public sphere is relatively affectless. Here the chief concerns are quality control, the attraction and maintenance of customer interest and the maximisation of profit margins. In this study, greater value was apparently ascribed, by both men and women, to the affective and aesthetic aspects of food preparation.

Hence, these findings question somewhat universalist assumptions, common in Western feminist analyses of housework (e.g. Oakley, 1979: Charles and Kerr, 1986), that domestic work has less value and is of lower status than paid work within the public sphere. According to such assumptions, equality between the sexes is judged according to the extent to which: (a) women participate in paid labour; and (b) men are involved in housework. The authority that Iranian women exercise in the domestic sphere highlights the need for more refined analyses of gendered relations and challenges orientalist stereotypes regarding the inferior and subjugated status of Muslim women. By their everyday provisioning within the family and by gifting and exchanges within their social networks, these Shi'ite Iranian women clearly derive considerable power and influence from their food-work.

The high status of domestic food-work appears to be related in particular to the importance attributed, by parents, to the appropriate feeding of their children and to the maintenance of their health and well-being. Parents were expressly concerned that their children should not lose their Iranian identity and many understood food (and language training) to be key means of instilling Iranian values, as described in Chapter 11. In their accounts parents often drew upon essentialist notions of culture in which their children were perceived to be ambiguously situated between two static and primordial cultural systems, pulled in two directions but belonging to neither (much of the health-related literature in Britain has also tended to represent ethnic minority youth in this way).

In fact, the food habits of these young people, as well as other consumption practices, such as choice of clothes, music and leisure activities, reflect a more flexible, 'pick n' mix' approach to the performance of ethnic and other transecting identities, such as those of gender, peer group, neighbourhood and class. Chapter 12 illustrates the multivocality and contingency of such affinities and considers whether such 'play' has lasting significance in the development of these young people's identities.

Drawing upon Bakhtin's distinction between organic and intentional hybridity (1981; 358), Chapter 12 also considers how the opposing culinary forces, towards novelty, on the one hand, and tradition, on the other are reflected through the food preparation and consumption practices of Iranian mothers and children. Within these Iranian families, children apparently function as the main culinary innovators, introducing and requesting new foods and recipes. Mothers, on the other hand, tend to act chiefly as stabilisers and moderators of change. Thus, domestic meal-planning and provisioning involves processes of negotiation and compromise between women and children, such that mothers may agree to incorporate novel dishes, provided their children also agree to eat Iranian food at other times. In their application of Iranian cooking techniques, herb and spice blends and serving modes, women maintain a sense of coherence and continuity. In so doing perhaps they also preserve a measure of ontological security, which may be necessary to the continuance of culinary 'play' among young people.

Finally, this text demonstrates what anthropology has to offer to our understanding of the complexity of meanings and uses of food within a particular sociocultural context. It highlights the disparate dimensions of this substance, which functions not only as the fuel which maintains vital physiological processes, but also as a marker of taste and identity, and as a commercial commodity which is implicated in prevailing political-economic relations. As I argue, food plays a central role in the construction and performance of identities, setting boundaries but also creating bridges between ethnic groups. Although food practices are responsive to change, at the same time they serve to maintain a sense of separateness and integrity. Ultimately, food is a social and aesthetic medium which for its consumers cannot easily or appropriately be broken down into its many components. An understanding of the significance of food in peoples' lived experience cannot then be adequately achieved by a rigid discipline-bound focus, such as that of nutritionists or of some social scientists. Rather, this text argues for and illustrates a more holistic and critical approach to the study of food and eating, an approach which encompasses political, economic and sociocultural analyses, and which acknowledges the significance assigned by men and women to the physiological aspects of food consumption.

2. ANTHROPOLOGICAL APPROACHES TO THE STUDY OF FOOD AND CONSUMPTION

Food holds a central place within the social order and for this reason it has long been a subject of considerable interest to anthropologists. Since the days of Mead (1943) attempts have been made to study the eating habits of selected populations. Often such observations were made as part of a wider ethnographic study of a specific population, but gradually a more specific interest in the anthropology of food emerged, leading to the eventual development of a distinct subfield of nutritional anthropology. A number of authors have undertaken reviews of the most significant perspectives to have held sway in anthropology and related disciplines, including Murcott (1988), Beardsworth and Keil (1997: 47–70) and Caplan (1997). It is not, therefore, my intention to reiterate each of these approaches in laborious detail, but rather, to consider what they may have to offer to contemporary researchers in the field of food and eating, and in particular how they might inform and enrich this study.

Functionalist Perspectives

Within functionalism, society is viewed as analogous to a living organism, composed of a set of interrelated features which maintain its cohesion and continuity. Particular institutions are then examined to determine their functional significance. During the formative years of the British school of social anthropology this approach was the dominant one. Ethnographies of 'primitive' social systems often including analyses of food systems; for example, Radcliffe-Brown's (1922) study of the Andaman Islanders examined the enactment of food rituals and use of taboos in relation to processes of socialisation. Malinowski focused more specifically on food production and allocation in the Trobriand Islands (1935) and he detailed the patterns of beliefs about food and modes of social reciprocity existing there. However, functionalism was widely criticised for failing to historicise institutions and focusing instead on their roles or effects. Additionally, its relatively static view of group social organisation, with its overemphasis on stability and continuity, was illequipped to analyse the external effects of change, with the result that this approach has been relegated to the margins of sociology and anthropology (Beardsworth and Keil, 1997: 60). Nevertheless, many of its ideas relating to food uses and practices have retained their salience; for example, Richards' analysis of the Bemba food system (1939) in the context of the wider economy, and her examination of the symbolic significance of food in 'cementing' ties of kinship, obligation and reciprocity. These themes remain highly pertinent in the present study, and are developed in Chapter 10. More importantly, with regard to this analysis (and contrasting starkly with the field of nutrition, in which nutrient intakes are commonly analysed as if eating is divorced from wider societal influences) functionalist perspectives view the food system, like society, in holistic terms, in which the interrelationships and interdependency of its component parts are seen to be important in shaping and characterising the overall system.

Structuralist Analyses

Structural approaches proceed from the recognition of the human capacity to deal in symbols and to assign significance to everyday objects, including food (Murcott, 1988). In contrast to the functional concern with the way in which various aspects of the social system interact to maintain a coherent whole, structuralists focus not simply on the 'surface' elements but on underlying or 'deep' structures reflecting the tendency of the human mind to construct binary contrasts (Jenks, 1993: 127; Beardsworth and Keil, 1997: 60). With the rise of structuralism in the sixties, the anthropological focus on food, particularly arising from the work of Lévi-Strauss, began to intensify (Caplan, 1997: 1). Food was analysed as a sign language which could be deciphered to reveal the underlying attitudes of the society under consideration. Study of food classificatory systems, the ways in which edible/inedible foods were differentially defined, the nature and logic of taboos, the sacrificial use of plants and animals and the social roles of food in exchange and commensality were some of the subjects examined by structuralists in order to analyse the particular ways in which humans imbue their social environment with meaning.

For structuralists, food was not so much the sustenance of organic life but, in Lévi-Strauss's famous aphorism, it was 'good to think' with. His aim was to decipher the rules and conventions governing food classification and preparation in order to comprehend the relationship between food systems and the social order. For example, in 'The Culinary Triangle' (1966) Lévi-Strauss examines cooking processes, which he argues, along with language acquisition, distinguish humans from other animals (see Figure 1). Thus, he emphasises how the cooking of food is important for its symbolic value and meaning (regardless of the physiological changes wrought). Borrowing methods of analysis from the field of linguistics, he applies the notion of oppositional relationships between phonemes (elements of language) to cuisines. He then identifies and associates a pair of binary oppositions – elaborated/unelaborated – according to which cooking represents a transformation and elaboration of the raw ingredients.

However, cooking is not the only means by which food can be transformed, it is also subject to rotting processes (and cooked food may also be subject to spoilage). Lévi-Strauss goes on to propose a second binary opposition – between nature and culture – which underlies this triangular semantic field. Thus he argues:

> the raw constitutes the unmarked pole, while the other two poles are strongly marked but in different directions: indeed, the cooked is a cultural transformation of the raw, whereas the rotted is a natural transformation. (Lévi-Strauss, 1966)

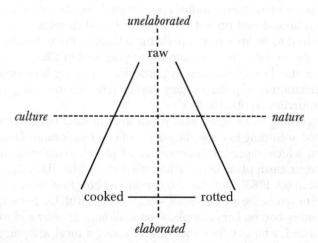

Figure 1 The culinary triangle; after Lévi-Strauss (1966).

Lévi-Strauss has been criticised for being more concerned with the structure of human thought than with food. Moreover, a number of authors have questioned the analytic and heuristic usefulness of his interpretation, particularly in his further elaboration of the culinary triangle, in which he considers specific cooking methods and their position relative to the basic triangle (Beardsworth and Keil, 1997: 62). Despite its limitations, and the rigidity of structuralism in demanding an analysis of systems of signification, this attention to cooking processes is an important consideration in the study of cuisines and will be further developed in subsequent chapters. However, in 'performing' my analysis of the food-work of Iranian women, I have eclectically recycled and applied elements of the culinary triangle, not in terms of a highly formalised structural analysis, but as pertaining to women's actual and variable culinary practices.

Mary Douglas was one of those influenced by Lévi-Strauss, although her work, issuing from the British anthropological school, is analytically and empirically Durkheimian. Douglas has made a substantial contribution to the study of food and eating, being particularly concerned with the ways in which food events serve as a microcosm of wider social structures and boundary definitions. In this way her structural approach to the study of food is integrated with her earlier work on ritual, taboo and pollution, and with subsequent consumption studies, illustrating that food habits cannot be divorced from the social context in which they occur. For example, early in her career Douglas undertook an analysis of Jewish dietary laws (as detailed in the book of Leviticus). She explained the dietary prohibition relating to pigs in the context of a classificatory system which defined these animals as anomalous (i.e. they are not cloven-hoofed and do not chew the cud) and therefore they were perceived to be impure and polluting (Douglas, 1970). Muslim food laws also prohibit the consumption of pork and in Chapter 6 I will pursue this line of analysis, in particular exploring how symbolic understandings of pollution may also be reflected in the organoleptic properties ascribed to foods.

According to Douglas, food is not food in itself but becomes so defined according to a specific system of communication. Thus, leftovers, which represent 'matter out of place', remaining on the no-longer-clean plate, become identified as inedible (Douglas, 1970: 48; Murcott, 1988). Douglas also considered how food can be understood to symbolise an individual's relationships with his/her self, and with other bodies. For example, what is allowed to enter and what is prohibited, who one feels comfortable eating a meal with, or, more intimately, sharing the same plate or cup with, 'speak' volumes about the order of everyday life. In one major study Douglas analysed the British diet, showing how it constitutes a particular 'system of communication' (1982). By examining the menu-composition and sequences of major and minor meals, and observing the scale of importance throughout the day, year and lifecycle, she demonstrated the apparent significance of how we eat, as well as what we count as food, arguing in this case for the symbolic importance of even the smallest food event (the biscuit) in representing the whole meal.

Douglas' work and that of other structurally-oriented social scientists remains crucial in illustrating the key role of culture in determining what and how we classify food and in beginning to comprehend the social and cultural meanings we ascribe to food. Nevertheless, it does little to explain changes in food habits or to decode the relations of power implicated in food systems.

Materialist/Developmental Approaches

A number of anthropologists and sociologists have observed that the focus on the symbolic overlooked the importance of social inequalities in determining access to food, as well as ignoring individual differences and economic and political influences. Materialist and developmental analyses take account of these factors and also have in common a focus on processes of social change, starting from the premise that in order to understand contemporary social relations and cultural forms an understanding of past forms is vital. For example, Mintz was concerned to demonstrate how historical, economic and political transformations impacted on the social significance of specific foodstuffs. In his case, the focus was on a single commodity – sugar. In *Sweetness and Power* (1985) Mintz explored the changing status of sugar within the culinary order, particularly over the last two centuries, and examined how the relationships between producers, plantation owners, slaves and the consuming public became bound up in the meanings of this substance. Hence, for him, the material aspects determining the availability of sugar within a geographical location and particular sociocultural setting inevitably precede its symbolic value and, moreover, must significantly influence those meanings.

Whereas some materialists were dismissive of the symbolic aspects of food consumption, Mintz's work engaged with their contributions, strengthening his own analysis. The physiological and sociocultural preference for sugar has resulted in it becoming a vehicle through which dominant sets of political-economic relations are played out internationally, modifying its symbolic meaning in a given context. It may then serve as an ideal organising metaphor for social relations in a particular society. In the following chapter I will examine some of the central meanings of sugar in Iranian society. Like Mintz, I integrate both symbolic and materialist perspectives; moreover, I will demonstrate how even our physiological responses to sweet foods are mediated by culture.

Mennell, a sociologist strongly influenced by the work of Elias, explored how changing social forces shape and modify food preferences and account for the evolution of specific cuisines. In *All Manners of Food* (1985) he considers the civilising of appetites of the English and the French and the development of their distinctively different cuisines, from the Middle Ages to the present. He analyses how the political transition from fuedal societies to modern states influenced and was reflected in major shifts in food consumption patterns and how cycles of feasting and fasting were ironed out as more constant food supplies were secured. In the process qualitative discrimination in food preferences became increasingly important as a marker of class and status.

Mennell also observes the impact of other cuisines upon British food culture. He argues that until the beginning of the twentieth century, British tastes were staunchly resistant to foreign influences (which he partly attributes to our puritan heritage). Then, however, French elements began to appear in the food culture of the upper classes, serving to mark their status and apparently resisted by the middle classes until well into the twentieth century. Since this time the influence of 'foreign' and increasingly of ethnic minority food cultures within Britain has grown, as I will discuss in Chapter 8 in relation to the relative invisibility of Iranian cuisine, and in Chapter 12 in a discussion of contemporary British culinary culture from the vantage point of Iranian youth. Ultimately Mennell argues that there has been a trend towards 'diminishing contrasts, increasing varieties' (1985: 321–32), such that across classes people have had greater opportunities for more varied experiences in eating and tastes in food. As a result, he asserts that there has been increasing uniformity of food practices throughout the social spectrum, although this has been contested by other observers, for example Warde (1997), as I will consider in the following chapter.

Harris, an American anthropologist whose theoretical approach is informed by sociobiological and ecological perspectives has, perhaps, been most dismissive of structuralist approaches to food consumption, arguing that the determinants of food-related behaviour are predominantly practical or are physiologically motivated (1986). Any symbolic element, therefore, needs to be interpreted according to nutritional, ecological and economic factors. For example, basing his argument on evidence that animal protein more closely matches human amino acid profiles and contains vital nutrients unavailable from plant sources, he attests that cross-cultural preferences for meat are related to human metabolic processes and requirements.

This type of approach has been very influential within the field of nutritional anthropology. The reductive, if not dismissive, response to the symbolic interpretation of food consumption is a major drawback of Harris's work, but he makes a valid observation that 'food must nourish the collective stomach before it can feed the collective mind' (1986: 15). The tendency of many anthropologists and sociologists to ignore or downplay the physiological aspects of food consumption is a limitation which will be addressed in the following chapter. The general public tend not to be so dismissive in this regard, and subsequent chapters illustrate how Iranian housewives attempt to balance their concerns to produce meals which are both nutritionally adequate and 'tasty' in aesthetic terms, as well as being culturally appropriate for particular occasions.

Food and Identity – Contemporary Approaches

Over recent years, anthropologists and sociologists undertaking research into food and eating have generally become less clearly affiliated with one particular theoretical school and more eclectic in their combination of historical, material and symbolic analyses. In terms of the research focus, they have tended to give increasing attention to the ways in which food serves as a marker of identity. Fischler, a French sociologist, is a key contributor in this area. He has been strongly influenced by structuralist approaches but shows marked affiliations to the developmental school – for example, he considers changes in the long-established rules, norms and meanings (i.e. rules of 'gastronomy') governing food systems. Fischler proposes that a state of 'gastro-anomy' (playing on Durkheim's concept of anomie) arises from the breakdown of those rules, in a climate in which the consumer is increasingly subjected to contradictory and inconsistent pressures (Fischler, 1980: 947; Beardsworth and Keil, 1997: 67).

In terms of his work on identity, Fischler argues that the symbolic value of food is so powerful that it comprises a major source of our sense of identity, at both an individual and group level (1988). He developed the principle of 'incorporation' to explain this process. Fischler points out that to 'incorporate' a food is, in both biochemical and ideological terms, to absorb all or some of its properties – 'we me what we eat' (Fischler, 1988). Combining a consideration of physiological and symbolic, the notion is of considerable value in a holistic analysis of food consumption practices as I found in interviews with respondents. It resonated powerfully with women's combined concerns as they engaged in their everyday domestic food-work to ensure the nutritional health and sociocultural wellbeing of their families.

Incorporation is the basis of collective identity and thus of marking a distinction from 'others'. A major way in which food delineates cultural identities is through the variable classification of edible and inedible items by different groups. There are many examples of foodstuffs valued in one culture but not considered edible in others – for example, horse meat is enjoyed in France but not eaten in Britain, and hedgehog, rejected by the ethnic majority is highly prized as a food by Traveller-Gypsies in Britain (Okely, 1983: 95). Pork, as I have already mentioned is forbidden to all Muslims, including Shi'ite Iranians. In addition to Douglas's observations in this regard, other explanations include Leach's contention that such avoidances may be related to how closely animals are conceptually linked with human societies (Leach, 1964). Those which are very distant, such as wild animals, or very close, such as pets, are taboo; hence although dog-meat is considered a delicacy in the Phillipines, the idea of eating 'man's best friend' is abhorrent in the U.K.

According to Fischler (1988), the relationship between food and group identity is two-way, in that the ingestion of certain foods not only leads to the incorporation of its associated symbolic value by the individual but also serves to assimilate the consumer into that particular culinary system. Data from this study accord with his assertion and women felt that they held a responsibility to feed their families with Iranian food (although the frequency of consumption required was variably interpreted) in order to ensure they retained their ethnic identities.

Whereas nutritionists have demonstrated considerable interest in the potential dietary problems associated with migration, Caplan (1997: 13) notes that there is relatively little social science data in Britain which directly considers the link between ethnic identities and food consumption, although the Medical Research Council unit in Glasgow is currently active in this respect, with ongoing studies of Irish, Italian and Pakistani settler groups there (M.R.C., 1996: 13–15). Additionally, anthropologists with other central concerns may also shed light on particular facets of food intake. For example, Werbner's (1990a) analysis of the symbolic meanings of British Pakistani wedding rituals and Gardner's (1993) exploration of the ties between homeland and diasporic Sylheti communities, expressed partly through food exchanges and gifting.

Although some degree of adaptation is to be expected according to the scarcity of traditional ingredients and the impact of dominant food cultures, nevertheless, the maintenance of familiar food habits may be of particular importance to migrants and may often act as a cohesive and stabilising force in a potentially alien environment (Kalka, 1988). Kalka, in her study of Gujarati settlers to Britain found that the evening meal in particular was most resistant to change, whereas breakfast, commonly not perceived to be a full meal, showed the greatest evidence of modification. Thus, her findings concur with Murcott's (1983) work on the significance of the cooked meal which I will discuss in the following section.

This text goes beyond these more tightly bounded works to seek an understanding of the multiple and diverse meanings of food within Shi'ite Iranian settler communities in Britain. Through inter-views with men, women and children, it explores the ways in which food figures in the daily lives of Iranian families, the power and influ-ence exerted through the giving of food within social networks, aspects of identity-formation through public food-work and beliefs about food and health. It shows how the family meal remains of cen-tral significance in reinforcing the emotional and relational ties within that unit, and observes how occasional celebratory communal events such as parties and picnics are particularly important in main-taining a sense of group cohesion.

The link between gender, food and identity is pursued more fully in Chapters 9 and 10. Briefly, however, it has been demonstrated that men and women have different rights of access to foods across cul-tures, with men commonly enjoying greater intakes of certain high status foods, such as meat and alcohol, as well as to larger servings. A number of researchers have closely examined the gendering of food provisioning and its implications (e.g. Murcott, 1983; Charles and Kerr, 1988; DeVault, 1991; Lupton, 1996). From this body of work common patterns emerge, in particular that domestic food-work is predominantly the responsibility of women and that they are heavily influenced by men's food preferences in their menu-planning. Although very valuable, these studies are all based on western popu-lations and are heavily influenced by western feminist perspectives regarding the interaction between gender and the apparently low sta-tus of domestic work, i.e., that women's domestic food-work not only reflects and expresses their subordinate status but also serves to rein-force it. As Beardsworth and Keil point out, the majority of these researchers rely predominantly on women's viewpoints and rarely incorporate men's or indeed children's first-hand accounts (1997: 86). Chapters 9 and 10 challenge some of these assumptions and illustrate how domestic food-work may provide an important, and sometimes jealously guarded, source of power for women.

Murcott has pointed out that in considering the importance of food in family life, the cooked meal, shared (ideally) by all family members, has carried and continues to hold particular symbolic valence (1982; 1983: 178–85; 1997: 32–46). Building upon Lévi-Strauss' analysis of the significance of the cultural transformations integral to the cooking process, Murcott argues that it is primarily the cooked dinner which signifies a 'proper' meal. Its production requires the application of heat through, for example, boiling or roasting (the latter method is essential to the preparation of the Sunday dinner, which comprises the cooked meal *par excellence*). Her analysis (1982) also integrates an elaboration of Douglas' work on the composition of the cooked meal, the vital elements (subject to geographic, historical and sociocultural variability) then being meat, potatoes, vegetables and gravy.

Data from this study accord with Murcott's key observations. In fact semantically the word 'food' is used by Iranians with reference to the cooked meal; it is this meal which has the greatest potential to symbolise 'the home, a husband's relation to it, his wife's place in it and their relationship to one another' (Murcott, 1983: 179). Of course, the elements necessary to constitute a proper meal differ from those identified in Murcott's study (as does the composition of contemporary British cooked meals, according to the increased variety of foods now available and current trends and fashions in food consumption). For many Iranians, rice is considered an essential component; in this case, stews containing mixtures of meat, beans, vegetables and herbs, rather than discretely prepared and served portions of each, predominate. Significantly, it is the cooked meal which is of key symbolic importance in the assertion of ethnic, national and religious identities, as will be explored in Chapter 6.

The performance of cooking and the production of the cooked meal by women can be further analysed in relation to the skills required and the emotional investment involved. Considering the aesthetics of home consumption, Leach (1998) draws on Csikzentmihalyi and Rochberg-Halton's (1981) 'The meaning of things' to consider the individual's active attempts to create meaning by the investment of psychic energy (interpreted in a behaviouristic and conscious way, rather than the Freudian sense) into ordinary objects, so enhancing their value and clothing them with 'an extra layer of meaning' in the process. In relation to food, Sered (1988) analyses the investment of physical, emotional and spiritual energy which is integral to the act of cooking. Examining the kitchen rituals of Middle Eastern Jewish women, she argues that the raw food becomes imbued with holiness, and the potential to strengthen relational ties, through the women's lavish and loving investment of time and energy during its preparation.

For secular women too, including these Iranian settlers, the process of cooking is one of transformation and enhancement, in which the sight, smell, taste and texture of the meal served 'speak' of the labour, love and expertise invested. Hence, the greater the investment of time, energy and skill into the dish, the greater will be the value of the final product and the standing of the cook in the eyes of its consumers. These aspects of meal provision and their implications with regard to the performance of gendered identities and power relations are pursued in Chapter 10.

Mauss first considered the importance of gifts in the creation and reproduction of social relationships (1950). The giving of food through exchange or gifting, everyday meals or dinner parties, provides women cross-culturally with a culturally sanctioned ability to attain influence through commanding reciprocal obligations, chiefly among family and friends (Counihan, 1988; Werbner, 1990a: 218–21;Theophano and Curtis, 1991: 148–49). The more lavish the food provided, and the greater the culinary efforts of the preparer, the greater will be the debt of obligation.

Psychoanalytic approaches offer further explanation for the construction of gender roles, evolving out of the primary feeding relationship, i.e. between the mother and child. According to this perspective, the mother's body not only represents sustenance and comfort but may also be a source of denial and frustration as she controls and restricts the infant's access to food and the comfort of bodily contact. Arising out of a Western worldview, psychoanalytical theories apply universalist notions in which autonomy and self-control are deemed to be normative processes in the construction of subjectivity. From this perspective, separation from the mother's body (with its ambivalent and leaky boundaries) and rejection of the nourishment and comfort associated with it are an essential part of individuation and maturation (Lupton, 1996: 45).

Fürst, following Chodorow, argues that it is the male (and in particular western male) who must construct his identity beyond the boundaries of his mother, by a severe separation from her. Thus she asserts that male identities are commonly very fragile and in need of constant reinforcement (Fürst, 1991: 127). Often the performance and reproduction of masculinity is secured by a series of denials of femininity, some of which are communicated through the medium of food. Through examples taken from 'primitive' societies, Fürst suggests that rules prohibiting men from cooking everyday meals, eating the same foods or at the same time as women thus serve to reinforce their personal boundaries (Fürst, 1991: 120). However, findings from this study suggest that in the case of non-western societies, where the process of individuation is not culturally sanctioned, masculine identities may be more robust and flexible. Hence, as I will explore in Chapter 9, it may be that Iranian men are able to perform tasks, including food-preparation, which are perceived to be women's work, without compromising their own identities. However, before engaging in depth with these ethnographic findings, the following chapter will further explore the social science contribution to the study of food, in particular considering how the recent analytical focus on the body has impacted upon research into food consumption.

3. FOOD, THE BODY AND TASTE

Recently, the body has become a major locus of interest within disciplines as varied as women's studies, literary criticism, history, comparative religion and philosophy (Csordas, 1994: 1). In sociology and cultural studies, the relationship between the body and consumption practices has increasingly been studied – for example, the ways in which commodities, including foods, and other goods, such as clothing and music, are used to obtain identity-value, encompassing style, status or group identification (Featherstone, 1991; Warde, 1996: 4–5; Falk, 1994). The current chapter considers the impact of this field of study upon our understandings of food selection and eating behaviour.

Food Consumption and Subjectivity

Lupton's recent text on this subject – *Food, the Body and the Self* (1996) – is an important contribution to the field, and is particularly valuable for its wide-ranging and interdisciplinary approach. Lupton draws upon the work of a number of social and cultural theorists, such as Foucault, Bourdieu, Elias, Douglas and Kristeva, as well as bringing together the empirical findings of a number of major sociological food studies over the last twenty years or so. Attention is given to the ways in which food discourses are presented in popular culture, medical and public health texts and to individual accounts of food preferences and habits, based on data derived from her own Australian studies. This combination achieves a holistic account of the intertwining of food behaviour, culture, embodiment and self in western societies.

Lupton views the body as a project which is in the process of becoming, through a process of continual refashioning. She employs

Foucault's concept of the 'practices' or 'technologies' of the self i.e. the ways in which individuals respond to external imperatives concerning self-regulation and comportment (1996: 15). These practices, which include food habits and preferences, are 'inscribed' upon the body, in culturally specific ways, for others to 'read' and interpret (Lupton, 1996: 140). For example, based on her own empirical data Lupton contends that dining out has become an increasingly important practice of the self in recent years, especially in western societies, the choice of restaurant and the food and drink selected offering the opportunity to construct and display different types of selves. Her line of reasoning offers a partial understanding of the relative lack of success of Iranian restaurants in this country. The perception and devaluation of Iranian cuisine and culture by British clients, aware of the negative stereotypes associated with the Iranian people may result in their reticence to be seen in these establishments, as will be explored further in Chapter 8.

Although in contemporary society the importance of the intentional manipulation of signs in the modification of individual identities has become increasingly important, the recent preoccupation in consumption studies with this fairly superficial process has tended to ignore deeper-rooted aspects of identity formation, more readily achieved through non-commodified processes linked with socialisation and group membership (Warde, 1997: 203). Warde's arguments, set out in his recent text – *Consumption, Food and Taste* (1997) are based on empirical research relating to changing representations of food and on reported eating practices.

Data were gathered from recipe features and advertisements appearing in a wide range of British popular magazines and from information derived from the Family Expenditure Survey, as well as from a questionnaire survey of households in the Greater Manchester region (1990). From these data, Warde identifies four pairs of long-standing structural oppositions which permeate the food and recipe columns: novelty/tradition, health/indulgence, economy/extravagance and care/convenience. These deep-rooted 'antimonies of taste', he argues, operate as powerful criteria for selecting foods, and are also applicable to other areas of consumption. Behind them, contends Warde, 'lie the structural contradictions that render problematic security, identity and belonging in late twentieth century Britain' (1997: 56).

Ultimately, his interpretation of the research findings leads Warde to contest Mennell's (1985) thesis which asserted that over the latter half of the century there has been 'increasing variety and diminishing contrasts' between the classes in terms of their food consumption practices. With respect to postwar Britain, Warde concedes that there

is now a greater variety of foodstuffs available to a much wider section of the population, largely as a consequence of the expansion of
supermarket chains. However, as he cogently argues, there is no evidence that such variety causes individuals to develop more diverse
sets of preferences. On the contrary, his findings regarding generational change suggest that younger cohorts have replaced previously
popular items with new tastes (1997: 167). Furthermore, Warde dis-
misses the applicability of Mennell's claim, primarily based on the
declining importance of class, for diminishing contrasts in food consumption patterns. Warde argues that any such decline occurred
after the war, in association with the disappearance of household
servants. In the late twentieth century, there is little evidence of class
contrasts diminishing, similarly differences of gender and generation also appear resistant to change (1997: 169).

Finally, counterposing contradictory stances between those, such
as Bourdieu (1984), who emphasise the importance of class expression and distinction expressed through group consumption practices,
and others, like Bauman(1990), who stress the importance of individual responsibility and the creation and definition of the self through
the use of commodities, Warde suggests that the extent to which the
role of commodity consumption figures in the formation of self-identity has been exaggerated. He argues that these have tended to focus
on consumer behaviour as if driven by processes of individualisation
and stylisation, whereas personal and social identities may be more
significantly and deeply impacted by noncommodified processes –
i.e., by acculturation and social learning in different contexts. Ultimately, an integrated approach to the study of food consumption
must give due consideration to both intentional and unconscious
aspects of the performance and transformation of identities. Such an
approach is undertaken here as will be more fully elaborated in
Chapter 12 in relation to the food intakes of young people.

The Body as Subject

Whereas early analyses of the body tended to privilege its objectivity – as a metaphor or text, or as a discourse to be cognitively understood – the phenomenological approach, such as that developing
from the work of Merleau-Ponty (1962) and latterly refined by Csordas (1994), highlights the importance of the sensory and perceptual
aspects of embodiment. Csordas seeks a more radical role for the
body, not simply as an object or theme of analysis, which takes
embodiment for granted, but as the 'existential ground of culture and

self' (Csordas, 1994: 6). Our bodies are not separate from ourselves, rather we *are* our bodies and we experience and understand the world through the synthesis of all our sensory perceptions. According to this perspective, the body, once seen as a fixed and constant biological entity, existing prior to the 'mutability and flux of cultural change and diversity' becomes an epitome of that flux (Csordas, 1994: 1–2). The implication is that our bodies, as beings-in-the-world, hold transformative powers over culture.

The phenomenological approach enables a more rounded understanding of the significance of food consumption. Food is a special substance, with the power to satisfy one of our greatest and most continual biological needs – the need to survive as a living organism. Although other consumer commodities may become 'meaningful extensions of embodied perception' (Leach, 1998) food physically enters the body, through the process of ingestion, passing through its boundaries (so that the body becomes open and vulnerable to the effects of food). Hence, it is associated with hope and anticipation but also with anxiety and danger.

Through psychosocial conditioning we learn to develop aversive behaviour in relation to taboo, unfamiliar or suspicious foods. This includes powerful emotive and bodily responses, such as discomfort, anxiety, sweating, nausea and retching. Data from this study offer empirical evidence to demonstrate the interweaving of social and biological aversive responses in the food consumption practices of Iranian settlers, as I will show in chapter . For example, non-*halal* meat is commonly perceived to have a tainted flavour, and pork is almost completely shunned by Muslim respondents. The capacity for overcoming innate aversions to unpalatable substances is also demonstrated to be culturally variable and often dependent upon early socialisation. Hence, in Chapter 12, I will demonstate that Iranian teenagers have commonly not developed a liking for alcohol, despite its widespread consumption (and the perceived pressure upon them to do so) by the ethnic majority.

Food and the Emotions

From the psychoanalytical perspective, the mother-child bond is seen to be a crucial factor in determining subsequent affective responses and desires associated with foodstuffs and eating. Like other cultural symbols, from early childhood food 'is embodied at multiple levels of consciousness' through the developmental processes (Lupton, 1996: 44). From infancy, through breastfeeding (and to an extent bottlefeeding), the close bodily contact between the mother and infant involves sensual pleasure and comfort, as well as nourishment, so that the infant comes to associate the assuaging of physical hunger with the reception of maternal love and the tactile reassurance of the mother's body. The sensory responses and meanings around feeding assimilated during infancy and childhood remain important in adult life and these contribute great potency to familiar and long-established food habits.

Clearly, food has the power to stir the emotions, both through its sensual aspects and its social meanings (Lupton, 1996: 31). Although novelists (for example Esquivel, 1993) have often explored these themes more successfully than social scientists, Lupton gives considerable weight to the importance of the emotions with regard to the experience of eating (1996: 30–36). One particular aspect she emphasises is the relationship between food and memory. Lupton argues that as an 'element of the material world which embodies and organises our relationships with the past in socially significant ways' food preferences share a symbiotic relationship with memory (1996: 32). The taste, smell or texture of a food or meal may trigger past memories, for example, for Guppy, an Iranian writer and exile living in Britain, the smell and sight of turmeric continues to evoke childhood memories in Iran of a blindfold horse shackled to a stone which ground the pungent spice.

> This is my first memory...a pungent, spicy smell wafts across the street; inside is a small dark room filled with clouds of yellow dust; in the middle a huge circular stone with a mast at its centre is being dragged round and round by a large emaciated horse on bending spindly legs. His eyes are blindfolded with a black cloth and, as he rotates the stone, a mustardy-yellow flour pours from under it into the surrounding gutter... The image dissolves. But it comes back, leaping into memory at odd times – in daydreams and nightmares, in moments of doubt and anguish, and every time I use turmeric in cooking: the skeletal blindfold horse, chained to its treadmill in a dark room, going round and round, day after day, year after year, all the while imagining that he is galloping in a daisy-dotted prairie, for a bag of oats at the end of the day. (Guppy, 1992:1–2)

The emotions aroused by foods may be strongly negative, ranging from disgust, anger and hatred, to more positive feelings of pleasure and desire. For many Iranians in this study the sight and smell of familiar food seemed to evoke nostalgic memories of home, family, security and contentment. It also brought reassurance about the love invested by the food provisioner and care-giver and the absence of familiar food sometimes led to profound emotive responses, as is most graphically illustrated in Chapter 11, by the account of one young boy separated from his mother.

Embodied Tastes

Lalonde (1992) in his analysis of taste and distaste, also attempts to demonstrate how our unspoken and embodied sensations and cognitive distinctions are interwoven according to specific sociocultural conditioning. The word 'taste' applied to food, commonsensically refers to its organoleptic properties (and a number of researchers have attempted to understand the physiological and biochemical mechanisms associated with the reception of flavours and aromas by the tongue and nasal sensory cells and to explain the variability in response according to changing substrate concentrations and ingredient profiles – for example, Scott and Giza, 1987: 28; Drewnowski and Schwartz, 1990). Alternatively, 'taste' has connotations (for sociologists and anthropologists in particular) of fashion and status. Bourdieu (1984) records the means by which the upper classes maintain their distinctiveness from the masses through the selection of specific food items, and James (1997: 77) describes how social tastes and trends in food consumption in contemporary Britain have changed as the elite seek new ways to reassert their status.

Influenced by the work of Merleau-Ponty (1962), Lalonde goes beyond structuralist analyses (such as Douglas's) of the 'meal-as-object' to a consideration of the 'meal-as-event'. Thus he sees eating as a lived experience which derives meaning from the complex array of sensory and cognitive factors involved (1992). Lalonde contends that in fact, it is very difficult to separate the organoleptic and symbolic aspects of taste, and that even the physiological perceptions of, and response to foods are socially conditioned. Thus an individual's taste, for example for a particular concentration of sugar, or its combination with other 'flavour principles' (as elaborated in Chapter 4), is inextricably linked with that of the group into which s/he is acculturated. Taste is then 'less a matter of *sensation* and more a matter of *perception* (his emphasis) i.e., the reception, cognition and interpretation of stimuli' (1992). Lalonde employs the term 'taste perception' which more accurately connotes the complex combination of physiological and symbolic responses occurring during each food event.

> (T)aste necessarily involves the participation of all our senses, thereby including the whole person...Furthermore if our cultural attitudes to food can override the normal functioning of our eating signals, does that not signify that taste is capable of joining forces with our symbolic constructions, contributing to the generation of insight? (Lalonde, 1992)

The possibility that culture can shape biological experiences and that our attitudes and conditioning may determine or override our sensory perceptions is a theme which is recurrent throughout this text. In this chapter the ways in which the taste for sugar is socioculturally and politically mediated serves as an example of that interrelationship. In subsequent chapters it becomes apparent that regional, national and global influences and identities are asserted through particular taste preferences and dominant 'flavour principles' and the capacity for modification, according to changing environments is explored.

The Sweet Tooth: Sugar as a Metaphor for the Food System and Wider Social Relations

Each of the approaches detailed in this and in the previous chapter have lent increasing weight to the notion that human eating behaviours and food preferences are profoundly influenced by sociocultural processes, and that anthropologists must take account of both macro and micro perspectives in order to give a comprehensive analysis of particular practices or processes. However, anthropologists must also recognise the physiological significance of food to its consumers. How do we address, for example, the universal and marked preference for sweet-tasting foods among human beings which, evidence strongly suggests, is based on the presence of an innate mechanism (Rozin, 1987: 101). Even postnatal infants have been demonstrated to prefer sweet solutions (and human breast milk contains high lactose loads). In fact, the preference appears to be more marked in childhood, although it persists throughout the lifecycle (Beardsworth and Keil, 1997: 242).

It has been suggested, according to materialist perspectives similar to those asserted by Harris (1986) that this preference has an ecological basis, that is, the sweet taste is characteristic of energy sources and is rarely associated with poisons (often identified by a bitter taste). Some psychobiologists have also argued that the preference for sweetness may offer the most clearcut illustration of the link between biology, individual and culture. For example, Rozin (1982: 228–29) contends that there is a straightforward progression between the innate physiological response and the development of behaviour patterns designed to seek out sweet foods. Once discovered, such items are readily incorporated into a cuisine; thereafter their existence in that food culture guarantees their exposure to future generations and the reinforcement of their edibility.

Without wishing to dismiss or ignore this line of argument, it is important to emphasise that the 'liking for sweetness, like that of every other sensory characteristic, is for a particular level in a specific, familiar context' (Booth et al., 1987: 146). Thus, although the physiologically mediated preference may be universal, the type of sweet foods consumed shows considerable crosscultural variation and the threshold for and interpretation of what counts as acceptably sweet is also culturally variable.

Significantly, the preference for sweet-tasting foods has provided the foundation of a transnational trade apparatus, geared to the production, manufacture and distribution of sugar and sweet foods (Beardsworth and Keil, 1997: 243–52). Mintz (1985) considered how the expansion of the cultivation of sugar cane became entwined with systems of world trade, colonial domination and the exploitation of slave labour. The human and economic price paid by sugar growing populations to satisfy the Western sweet tooth is also considered in Scheper-Hughes' *Death Without Weeping* (1993), an evocative account of poverty, malnutrition and infant mortality in contemporary Brazil. Thus contemporary nutritional judgements of sugar as 'pure white and deadly' (Yudkin, 1972) according to its implication in the aetiology of dental caries, obesity, coronary heart disease and diabetes mellitus, may also be understood to incorporate more deep-rooted symbolic meanings.

As previously mentioned, Mary Douglas has argued that within the British meal system the biscuit is capable of acting as a condensed symbol, standing for 'all the sequences of puddings throughout the year and of wedding cakes and christening cakes throughout the life-cycle' (1982: 97). Given the importance of the innate cross-cultural preference for sweet foods and additionally, the scale of development of the sugar trade, as well as the gross inequities in the political-economic relations of power intrinsic to its evolution, this substance clearly has the propensity to serve as a metaphor for both food in general and the food system more widely, encompassing processes of production and consumption.

Sweet or Sickly? Taste as the Embodiment of Culture

Within British culinary traditions, there are strong predilections for cakes, puddings and confectionery, but relatively few sweet ingredients appear in everyday main courses. Their relegation to the end of the meal or to between meal snacks, or their addition to food in the form of condiments, such as ketchup and chutney, may be related to the considerable ambivalence regarding sugar and sugar-containing foods in our society. On the one hand, these foods are associated with pleasure and satisfaction, yet on the other hand with guilt and fear (exacerbated by nutrition and health education messages).

Once ascribed medicinal properties, sugar is still used in the production of pharmaceuticals, but only as a 'filler' or to mask bitter-tasting drugs. In dietary terms it has been demoted from its former, highly esteemed status; now labelled 'empty calories', sugar hovers on the fringes of nonfood, or even poison, with its 'pure white and deadly' image. Ironically, fructose ('natural' fruit sugar), maltose (a derivative of raw sugar), molasses, raw cane sugar and honey (the ultimate 'natural' sweet food) are all currently ascribed certain healthgiving properties. James (1990) asserts that the marginal status of sweet foods (and in particular confectionery), viewed in terms of their structural integration within the meal cycle, and their ambiguous status between food and nonfood, actually enhances their capacity to act as symbolic currency. Thus she contends that chocolate serves as the ideal gift, expressing love and appreciation, particularly at Christmas and Easter. Reed-Danahay (1996) has further explored the symbolic potential of chocolate, in this case its significance in the wedding rituals of rural Auvergne. Mixed with champagne and served in a chamber pot, it thus symbolises human waste, so temporarily overturning everyday practices of acceptable behaviour and challenging class-based attitudes regarding taste and high culture.

Within Iranian cuisine there are very different uses and meanings ascribed to sugar and sweet-tasting foods, which arise out of, and intersect with, historical and political-economic influences governing availability and access, as well as different cosmologies. For example, sugar, especially in the form of *nabat* (rock sugar), is still perceived to have medicinal properties; within the humoural framework it is considered to counteract cold conditions as is illustrated in Chapter 5. Hence, its consumption retains positive health connotations. This may partially explain why Iranians use sweet ingredients more widely as an intrinsic part of the main course, where it comprises an integral element of some of the dominant 'flavour principles'. In contrast, desserts and cakes tend to be reserved for special occasions.

There also appear to be major discrepancies between English and Iranian perceptions of sweetness. Iranian tastes for sweet foods apparently privilege syrupy or sweet-starchy mixtures, often with very subtle hints of other flavours, such as cardomom or saffron. To British palates these may be considered sickly sweet (and as discussed in Chapter 8, some Persian restaurant owners acknowledged that this course was the least appealing element of the meal to British customers). Although it might be expected that the presence of fruit, acid and fat would result in a reduced perception and greater tolerance of high sugar loads, to Iranian palates 'rich' mixtures, such as

Christmas cakes (even those containing no alcohol and consumed without the icing) are commonly thought to be too sweet. The very richness, often perceived by British palates to compensate for or to counterbalance the sweetness, seems for many Iranians to contribute to sensory overload and distaste (and perhaps underscores the lack of subtlety they commonly associate with British food tastes). However, many of the younger generation (often familiarised through the school meals system) did appear to have developed more anglicised tastes and some were very partial to English cakes and puddings. In this regard, as was more generally evidenced in their diets (as will be examined in Chapter 12), significant shifts and 'play' with food cultures appeared to reflect wider transformations in cultural identities.

Perhaps it may also be that the sickliness we (especially middle class) British perceive in consuming sugar is a consequence of our own acculturation. Contemporary health connotations may explain why, beyond a certain concentration (variable according to individual, gendered and status-related taste thresholds), sugar seems to taste sickly to us – we may harbour deep-rooted anxieties that it will indeed make us sick. However, for Iranians it seems to be the richness of cakes and puddings, perhaps associated with anxiety over the health risks of a high fat intake which is perceived as too (i.e., unpleasantly/unhealthily) sweet.

In addition to its medicinal use, sugar also provides a key ingredient in the drinking of tea, a habit elaborated in a specific way and thus one means by which Iranian identities are clearly marked and reinforced (Harbottle, 1995: 27). Lump sugar is held between the teeth, and the tea, which is served black, is sipped through it. In Britain, Iranians are generally obliged to buy commercially processed sugar cubes, as *nabat* (rock sugar) is not readily available. However, these quick-dissolving cubes are not wholly suitable as they release too great a concentration of sugar, too quickly. Even the simple performance of drinking tea in Britain therefore involves a subtly different taste experience for Iranian settlers, and expresses not simply a reassertion but also marks a slight transformation in cuisine and cultural identities, which resonates powerfully within the diet as a whole.

The taste for black tea served with sugar carries additional significance among the older generation of Shi'ite Iranians. According to one informant, during the fifties the short-lived government led by Mossadegh (a national hero and opponent of the former Shah's oppressive rule) challenged British control of Iranian sugar (as well as petroleum sales) with enormous popular and clerical support. When public demand was ignored by the British, religious leaders precipitated a downturn in sugar sales by declaring it *haram* (effectively forbidding its consumption by Muslims). When an agreement was finally reached and the government wanted to restore sales, the new taxonomic categorisation became a problem. A solution was suggested by one of the religious leaders; it was declared that if the sugar was dipped into liquid before consumption, it could be made acceptable once more. This neat manoeuvre not only solved a material problem but as my informant pointed out 'no-one else drinks tea like that'. Thus, the specific manner of incorporation here serves to distinguish Iranian Muslims, not only from non-Muslims but also from Sunnis, and, by continuing to drink their tea in this manner, even in Britain, these Iranians reassert their Shi'ite identity.

Among some exiles, there is perhaps yet another layer of meaning to be registered in seeking an understanding of the significance of this practice. Some of those interviewed expressed high regard for the integrity and courage of Mossadegh, one of the few political figures (prior to Khomeini) who risked his life by seeking justice and freedom from western interference. There was a strong feeling amongst many Iranian exiles (also expressed by Farman Farmaian with Munker, 1992: 271–77) that, had he not been assassinated, the revolution could have been avoided. In continuing to drink tea with lump sugar therefore, some Iranians may also symbolically engage with his resistance to the pervasive influence of western political and cultural influences. This theme and the notion of 'west-toxification' will be further pursued in subsequent chapters, in particular Chapter 6.

The foregoing account illustrates how even in a microanalysis of one particular foodstuff, or of a single taste preference, the political, economic and social contexts impinge upon, shape and transform the symbolic understandings of, and the physiological responses to a substance. Thus the need for a holistic perspective in the study of food and eating is evident. It is equally important that any analysis of food consumption takes into account indigenous cosmologies of food and health. Since Iranians themselves take a holistic view of diet and health, it is clearly inadequate to apply only, for example, a structural analysis to their patterns of food consumption. While the following chapters particularly emphasise the symbolic dimensions of food consumption among Iranians in Britain, this approach is complemented by, and interwoven with a consideration of the political, economic and social currents which have moulded British Iranian food culture. Moreover, this analysis recognises and explores the lay nutritional knowledge of Iranian settlers and how they perceive the incorporation of food to affect their bodies and their wellbeing.

4. 'NUTRITIOUS AND DELICIOUS'
IRANIAN WOMEN AND THEIR DOMESTIC FOOD-WORK

During the preliminary field work it had become apparent that the everyday food preparation tasks of Iranian women were perceived to be very important and were valued by themselves and their families accordingly. This contrasted sharply with the low status held by those men who were employed in the catering trade (as will be discussed in Chapter 7). Moreover, the respect accorded to Iranian women at home appeared to be dissonant with more generalised stereotypes pertaining to Muslim gender roles.

The following chapters focus on the nature and definition of women's domestic food provisioning in order to understand why it is perceived to be high status work. This is shown to be related to its function as an integral element of daily healthcare and to its symbolic significance in the maintenance of ethnic identity. In interviews with women it was apparent that they had two predominant concerns in the daily provision of food for the family, the first was to provide a nutritionally adequate and healthy diet (as will be considered in the next chapter) and the second was to ensure that meals were tasty and aesthetically pleasing to their families. This chapter considers the dual meaning of the term taste and demonstrates how national, regional, global and local cultural influences and identities are performed through specific food consumption practices. It also considers the significance of women's aesthetic work in ensuring the emotional wellbeing and sociocultural stability of the family.

Iranian Cuisine: Regional and National Taste Preferences

In nutrition parlance the word 'taste' tends to be applied to the organoleptic properties of food, i.e., the physiological sensations associated with the aromas and flavours perceived by the tongue and nasal sensory cells of an individual; to social scientists it carries connotations of style and status. However, as the empirical examples in this text demonstrate, the physiological and symbolic aspects of taste are not so easily separated. Rather, organoleptic responses may be significantly moulded by sociocultural conditioning. Hence, taste may be 'less a matter of *sensation* and more a matter of *perception,* i.e. the reception, cognition and interpretation of stimuli' (Lalonde, 1992, original emphasis). Lalonde's term 'taste perception' usefully connotes the complex combination of physiological and symbolic responses occurring during each food event and it is adopted here in the exploration of national, regional, global and local culinary tastes and their relevance in the performance of ethnic identities.

Food 'shares its part-instrumental part-aesthetic place in the range of all art forms with clothing, architecture and utensil design' (Douglas, 1982: 106). Like Persian art, crafts and literature, the high cuisine of Iran is sophisticated, elaborate, colourful and rich, with a complex and subtle blend of herbs, spices, fruits and nuts; everyday meal preparation is also a complex matter. Within Iranian food cultures there are key dominant taste themes or 'flavour principles' (Rozin, 1978: 105; Lalonde, 1992) which may be considered to be the principal signifiers or most characteristic elements of that food culture. For example, 'sweet-sour' and 'sweet-savoury' combinations are prevalent throughout the country, as are varied and distinctive combinations of meat with beans/nuts, herbs/spices and fruit. The distinctive fruit/meat combinations can be traced back to pre-Islamic times, hence they may symbolically represent a perpetuity and stability of culinary identity, in opposition to the political upheaval and change which has taken place, especially in recent history (Fragner, 1994a: 55).

Among Iranian settlers in Britain, considerable continuity is demonstrated with regard to cooking methods and preference for familiar taste themes. Certain ingredients, such as dried limes, pomegranite juice, *sumac* (an astringent powder), various herbs, and nuts are essential for this purpose. Although many of these items are available locally, sometimes from Iranian-owned stores, products brought from Iran are preferred. Women (generally the procurers of these products) often justify their choices on grounds of taste 'You can buy them here but they taste funny ....' (Soraye). Although the soils, weather and other growing and storage conditions do have important effects on the organoleptic properties of food, it seems that in this case the physiological response is also influenced by psychological and sociocultural conditioning (for a further discussion of this point see Harbottle, 1995: 36).

'In Iran every city has its own culture (and food) and if you travel you feel the difference from your home' (Mahmood). Within the shared (and extensive) vocabulary of national dishes and themes (Zubaida, 1994a: 34), regional distinctions also continue to be expressed by Iranians in exile. Partly, regional food characteristics have arisen as a result of different geographical influences, so that some ingredients have been available only in certain areas. In regions bordering the Caspian sea and in the southern Gulf provinces, fish is plentiful, hence local cuisines reflect the dependence upon fish products, although in these two regions, disparate in climatic conditions and ethnic composition, very different styles of fish cookery have evolved (Zubaida, 1994a: 35).

Although to many Iranian settlers rice is an essential element of a 'proper' meal, traditionally its cultivation has been restricted to small areas. In most parts of Iran, a meal without bread is unthinkable (Zubaida, 1994b: 93). A woman from Mosandan, a rice-growing area distinguishes her own customs from those of her husband (from Kerman), illustrating how different key elements are required to satisfy regional tastes.

> Mehri[1] – When I eat rice, I don't eat bread, just sometimes, but my husband, he has to eat rice and bread together (or) he feels hungry again.

The sweet-sour flavour principles form a dominant theme throughout the country but the preference for the sour element is stronger in some areas, for example in Teheran and central Iran, people are particularly keen on *qurut* – black fermented yoghurt, which is eaten as a snack, in the same way as nuts. Dried pressed plums are also popular here. Use of some spices is also specific to certain areas and hot spicy dishes are preferred in the southern provinces.

> Safieh – Sometimes I cook for my husband (who is from Abadan) for example – samosa …he likes samosa and *galie* …*khoresht* – but with fish, vegetables and tamarind. And its very spicy and they eat this kind of *khoresht* with *polou* rice … (like) Arabic food.

Differences in taste preferences were employed by interviewees to define ethnic boundaries and to assert superiority over settlers from other provinces. For example, the differences between the cuisine of Azerbyjan and other regional tastes were commonly mentioned. Azeri cooking, especially that of Tabriz, holds an especially high reputation (Zubaida, 1994a: 34). Although the region has linguistic affinities with Turkey, the food tastes noticeably Iranian, but with its own distinctive features (Fragner, 1994a: 54). Azeris are considered to use more lemon juice and butter in cooking than other Iranians and are reputed to take meticulous care over the preparation and presentation of dishes. Some women (particularly outsiders who had married Azeri men) aligned themselves with that ethnic group by adopting their style of cooking and by referring positively to the delicious taste of the food. In contrast, others (some of whom had also intermarried) maintained their own regional affinities, simultaneously considering Azeri cuisine to taste inferior to their food.

> Hamideh – They (Turks) are ...very patient ...in cooking, they're very careful ...especially they're really fussy about rice but to be honest ...I think – you know *ghormesabzi*.? ...I don't think Turkish people make it as good as it should be. They're good at ... *kofte Tabrizi*, you know, and I think ...they are very particular about *dolmeh* ... My mother-in-law has very small pieces of ...vine leaves ...and spends a lot of time. And she was a teacher, she was working. I mean she would do that at weekends ... They spend a lot of time on cooking and are ... very particular about it but I think ...they don't know about ...most of the foods that are particularly ...known as Iranian food ... You know, most of the *khoreshes* ... But anyway they are very particular about everything and they are famous for it and they are famous for cooking ....

It has been suggested that, symbolically, an individual's mouth may be regarded as a gateway by which that person guards and protects the self from the outside (Fischler, 1988; Falk, 1994: 14: Lupton, 1996: 18). By extrapolation, the capital city of a country also stands as the gateway and entrance point of that nation to the rest of the world. With regard to Teheran, the cosmopolitanism of the Iranian capital city and openness of its inhabitants to new and varied tastes in regional and international foods (and to new fashions generally) was positively stressed by some exresidents and contrasted with the unsophisticated and limited culinary repetoire and the narrow-minded outlook of those from the provinces. However, in the eyes of some migrants, this openness represents a danger; many Teheranis have been so influenced by foreign cultures and cuisines that they have lost their identity as 'true Iranians'. Hence, a discriminating palate may be seen to act as a protective mechanism against personal and cultural contamination.

Incorporation, Taste and Identity

Certain dishes, incorporating dominant taste themes and key ingredients, apparently hold particular valence in enabling an individual to *feel* Iranian and to be more powerfully drawn into the group; the different smells, textures and tastes, becoming 'inescapably embedded in the individual psyche' (Sered, 1988). In this study, one of the most commonly mentioned of these was *ghormeh-sabzi*, a stew composed of lamb, beans, vegetables and herbs.

Safieh – Some foods are basic, everyone likes, for exam
…because I think it's our traditional food and everywher‹
but maybe there is some little difference. For example, my
like red beans in *ghormeh-sabzi* but my husband likes the (l

Although *ghormeh-sabzi* is consumed throughout Iran, d‑‑‑‑‑‑ styles
of cooking, and/or slight variations in the ingredients, have served to
mark different regional identities; for example, apart from the use of
different types of beans, there may be variation in the type and
amount of fat used, in the quantities and proportional contributions
of the herbs and limes, and contestation over whether tomatoes
should or should not be included. In Britain, the dish becomes an
appropriate medium by which to represent the multivalency of Iranian identity, according to regional, ethnic, religious and family backgrounds, reflected in subtle alterations to the basic recipe. It is also
symbolic of positive incorporation, i.e. of safety and of self, as such
it has the power to (re)incorporate the eater into Iranian cuisine, culture and cosmology.

As described previously, incorporation is the action in which we
'send food across the frontier between the world and the self' (Fischler, 1988). It is a basis of identity; to ingest food is to incorporate all
or some of its properties. Hence, we become what we eat: (a) as nutrients are used in the synthesis of new tissue and to maintain vital metabolic processes; (b) as the symbolic characteristics of food are
absorbed and shape our individual and collective identities. Therefore, we are able to manipulate the diet and to remake ourselves, both
metabolically and symbolically, that is, to increase or decrease body
size and to boost our immune systems, or to retain, modify or transform our individual and/or collective identities. Fischler poses the
question: 'If we do not know what we eat, how can we know who we
are?' (1988) In the case of migrants, and in particular these Iranian
settlers in Britain, I propose that one of the chief means by which they
are able to determine and define who they are is through the performance of specific food preparation and consumption practices.

Changes and Continuities in Tastes: Local and Global Influences

Many interviewees have continued to consume Iranian food on a regular basis. For them, the British diet does not satiate their appetites,
rather, consumption of Iranian food, with its familiar taste and associated symbolic value, is apparently vital, not only to nourish the body,
but to satisfy the psyche and to strengthen the social body.

> Goli – When I have Iranian food …I am not any longer hungry …it sat-
> isfies me but with English food I am not satisfied … I'm looking for some-
> thing else …especially with rice, I have to eat rice.

Nevertheless, women are obliged to rely predominantly upon British ingredients and it was acknowledged by some informants that the taste of these cooked dishes is subtly different (Harbottle, 1995: 36). Even among those who had spent many years in Britain, some continued to perceive the flavour of meals in Iran to be superior to those dishes prepared here. In other cases, informants noted a change in their taste perceptions such that one woman found that she no longer liked the flavour of food prepared by her mother, but preferred her own culinary efforts, based on British ingredients (Harbottle, 1995: 36). Significantly, this woman also admitted that she could no longer consider returning to Iran to live and now thinks of England as her permanent home, illustrating how shifts in ethnic (and other) identities are powerfully reflected through tastes in food. The tension between the contrasting tendencies within cultures and cuisines towards continuity on the one hand, and change on the other, described by Warde (1997: 57) as the 'culinary antinomy of novelty and tradition', will be further considered in Chapter 12 .

Global influences upon food preferences, mediated predominantly through travel experiences, the media and education, were apparent in the eating habits of most interviewees. For example, the account of one informant illustrates particularly clearly the impact of different cultural influences in the evolution of her present multifaceted eating habits. In Teheran, her father owned a very successful international restaurant, hence she had become accustomed to developing new tastes in food from an early age. After marrying, she and her husband moved to Italy and they experimented freely with the local cuisine. Her present diet incorporates strong Italian and Iranian themes, and is further expanded by other international recipes gleaned from television. As in the case of other Iranians, her incorporation of British cuisine is limited, in this case to the occasional consumption of fish and chips. Significantly, in the syncretic process, Fatimeh's response to some Iranian foods has changed. For example, in Iran spaghetti is served in a distinctive manner, i.e., with *tadik* (a special potato or bread crust) and is very popular. However, Fatimeh now finds that she dislikes this dish and prefers spaghetti cooked in the 'proper' Italian fashion.

Another woman had spent several years in the U.S.A. (and had adopted certain aspects of that fast-food culture) before finally settling in Britain. Currently her food preferences are also strongly influenced by health concerns (according to the knowledge she has gleaned from studying as a beautician) as well as an emphasis on convenience foods, unusual among the Iranians interviewed. Iranian food retained a residual but important role within her diet, being reserved mainly for special occasions.

> Monir – (We don't eat Persian food) very often because we think that, especially in the evening, it tends to be a bit heavy and um with Persian foods, because they're *so tasty*, you tend to eat a lot … .(my emphasis)

As in the case of many of the women, for Monir, it seemed to be the special events, such as picnics and parties, where the use of Iranian food held particularly powerful valence in terms of maintaining identity (see Harbottle, 1995: 30 for a further discussion of this point). For Iranians generally, the offering of food is an important signifier of hospitality, acceptance and friendship; even if unexpected visitors arrived, mounds of fruit, sweets (such as nougat) and dishes of nuts would be presented.

> Soraye – In Iran, when the guests come, after they say hello to each other, they don't ask, 'would you like tea/coffee', they never ask, they go and get …and after that, maybe you don't have fruit in the house, doesn't matter, whatever you have – pistachios (etc) they bring and they insist, 'please you help yourself' …if you don't offer it, it is rude … .

This study is particularly concerned with everyday food consumption practices, but celebratory food events, both religious and secular, were commonplace and of great significance. For example, as well as the lavish provision of food at parties (Harbottle, 1995: 24–30), other cultural and religious events, such as *No Ruz, Moharram,* and *Charsamburi,* also incorporated the serving of specific special foods. Even more frequently, picnics and barbecues and regular informal, spontaneous meals offered the opportunity for the performance of ethnic (and gender) identities, through specific provisioning and consumption practices. These social gatherings were apparently highly significant means of maintaining the wellbeing and integrity of the family (and wider community).

For expatriate Iranians, trips to Iran are highly important events for the reaffirmion of cultural identity and the reinforcement of family ties (Harbottle, 1995: 34–36). Throughout such visits, food provides a powerful vehicle to communicate the care of the host relatives (and may serve as a means of expressing dysphoric affect). During the stay, family members prepare for the impending separation and return of the visitors to Britain. As part of this process, food supplies are gathered and prepared (with the investment of a considerable amount of labour) which will serve to maintain kinship and cultural ties until the next visit. The specific items chosen to maintain links may be those instrumentally considered unobtainable, expensive or of inferior quality in Britain. Significantly, they are often those marginal substances particularly valued for their medicinal and restorative properties, a point I will return to in the following chapter. Many are of key symbolic value, in that they are essential for the preparation of Iranian dishes, for example, saffron, dried limes, *sumac, zeresht* and herb mixtures are used in cooking; others, such as the nuts and sweets offered to guests, serve individually as ethnic markers.

> Soraye – …pistachios, …the nougat (sweets), …I always bring 2–4 kg and finish (the) first one in first few days! ….Dried (limes) definitely. My mother makes them, ….*zeresht* (small red sour berries) definitely, almonds and pistachios, walnuts – you can buy them here but they taste funny – they are not as fresh. When you buy them fresh they are a bit sweet, …*sumac* for *chelo kebab* and – I use lots of dried mint – and (my mother) she … dries it.

Food Preparation as a Means of Maintaining the Wellbeing of the Family

For Iranians, as for other groups, meal provision and commensality are vital in maintaining emotional wellbeing, spiritual harmony and in reinforcing cultural identity, as well as ensuring good nutritional status. These dimensions are also recognised by the World Health Organisation (W.H.O., 1982) as necessary to the maintenance of good health, nevertheless in many quarters, and particularly within the biomedical discourse, health still tends to be perceived in terms of an absence of organic disease. A pervasive, Western, mind/body dualism is reflected in the semantic distinctions between 'health' and 'wellbeing', the latter being considered to comprise (less valued) emotional and material influences. In Iranian cosmology, no such dualism exists, rather, there are powerful links between environmental factors, the emotions and the body. Frankenberg (1986) has suggested the use of an alternate term – 'well'th' – which encompasses consideration of material influences and effectively overcomes the 'health'/'wellbeing' divide. In this text I have adopted his term to more accurately conceptualise the concerns of Iranian families and in particular the food-provisioning responsibilities of these women.

This chapter has begun to consider how the aesthetic aspects of domestic food production are important in maintaining a sense of Iranian identity and in ensuring the wellbeing of families within the diaspora. As in most cultures, it is the women within settler Iranian communities who are largely regarded as responsible for the day-to-day provisioning of food, for guarding the health of their families and for treating sickness through the preparation of special foods, herbal remedies and other medicinal treatments. In the following chapter I will explore how women syncretically combine traditional and biomedical understandings of nutrition and health, illustrating how the physiological and cultural aspects of consumption are closely intertwined.

Note

1. Pseudonyms are employed throughout this text.

5. FOOD AND HEALTH
TRADITIONAL AND MODERN INFLUENCES

This section further examines Iranian women's domestic food-work. It highlights the holistic approach taken to healthcare within Iranian cosmologies and focuses on the interlinkages between diet and daily health maintenance, in particular the importance of hot-cold beliefs. It explores the relative influence of traditional beliefs and biomedical precepts in women's roles as the guardians of health within their families and illustrates the pervasiveness of biomedical models. Although many women considered themselves to have abandoned traditional thinking, the significance of balance within the diet remains very strong. The enmeshing of physiological and cultural concerns was further demonstrated in interviews by the use of nutrition and health discourses in the construction and reinforcement of national, regional, generational and educational identities.

Traditional Concepts

In Iranian cosmologies all aspects of life style influence health status, and ideologies of individual and social health invoke concepts of balance, harmony, integration and wholeness. Traditional beliefs are based on Galenic-Islamic medical principles, elaborated by Ibn Sina, from Arabic, Greek, Latin and Indian philosophies. Within this system individual temperament is believed to be derived from a distinctive balance of the four humours and their associated properties (blood – hot and moist; red bile/bilious – hot and dry; phlegm/serous – cold and moist; black bile/atrabilious – cold and dry). Temperament is considered to be variable according to age, sex, race and climate (Pliskin, 1987: 135–36). The body is also believed to be physically sensitive to elements within the environment and at certain stages in the life cycle, such as early childhood, individuals are particularly susceptible to alterations in climatic conditions.

Diet (through the notions of hot and cold – *sardi-garmi* – foods) interacts with climatic influences and individual temperament to affect health. 'Hot' or 'cold' qualities (referring not to thermal temperature but to perceived intrinsic properties) are ascribed to body conditions, foods, and medicines. Proper bodily function of an individual is maintained through consumption of a diet balanced in relation to intake of foods with these qualities. Illness is perceived to be caused by an imbalance in the hot/cold equilibrium, and results in specific reactions such as digestive problems, skin eruptions, sore throats and headaches (Pliskin, 1987: 140). This can be rectified through consumption of foods with opposing qualities and/or specific medicinal treatments.

Theoretically, then, health is maintained by an active and constant process of balancing one's body base, which demands daily attention to food consumption. Equilibrium encompasses a range of states, as individuals have different bases, according to inherited characteristics, birth circumstances, sex, season and lifestage. The action of diet, drugs, tonics, herbs and the environment all influence the equilibrium. The base state of children is regarded as 'hotter' and less stable than that of adults and they tend to be more susceptible to 'hot' illnesses (Pliskin, 1987: 137). Men usually have 'hotter' bases than women, and they demonstrate a greater degree of tolerance to changing conditions.

A large body of research exists, identifying different frameworks based on humoural principles (impacting on food and health ideologies) throughout the world (e.g., Greenwood, 1981; Messer, 1981; Tan and Wheeler, 1983). Those operating in the Middle East, Europe and the 'New World' are believed to be derived from the Galenic system; parallel systems apparently exist in the Far East, Southeast and South Asia (Messer, 1981). Although the general structural principles may be shared worldwide, there are significant variations in the detail and practice of these systems both within and between cultures (Greenwood, 1981; Tan and Wheeler, 1983). For example, in formal Ayurvedic and Chinese systems, the 'hot-cold' distinction is the major idiom for discussing moral, social, and ritual states, in addition to the specific qualities of foods and medicines, yet at folk level, only discrete elements of these beliefs may be adhered to and these may be interwoven with other concepts (both traditional and modern) relating to food and health. Similarly, in Morocco, elements of the Galenic humoral system have been integrated with Islamic medicine in present day pluralist practices, and a wide degree of intracultural variation in classifying foods has been demonstrated, according to personal knowledge and experience (Greenwood, 1981). Meanwhile, in Japanese popular health beliefs, only remnants of the 'hot-cold' framework remain, consisting of pairs of foods which are thought to cause food poisoning if consumed together (referred to as *kuiawase)* for example, mushrooms and spinach (Lock, 1980: 97).

Migration and Syncetism

Research by nutritionists and medical sociologists among migrant groups in Britain has tended to proceed from an applied perspective, in which it is hoped that knowledge of traditional beliefs will enhance the provision of health education and/or meal provision within state-run institutions. In the current study, establishing the importance of hot-cold beliefs offered a useful and nonthreatening starting point in interviews, from which to explore wider influences upon consumption patterns and food-work. According to the existing literature, maintenance of traditional practices may vary according to level of education, as well as prior exposure and current knowledge of traditional and alternate belief systems, such as biomedicine. For example, Chinese mothers in London reportedly maintain a high level of regard for their traditional practices, even if they feel constrained, and prevented from fulfilling their requirements, by environmental circumstances (Tan and Wheeler, 1983). Second generation Punjabi women in Glasgow are apparently more variable in their adherence to hot-cold beliefs (Bradby, 1995) but seem to retain a reasonable level of knowledge concerning them. However, the majority of women interviewed in this study declared themselves to be sceptical (a few were completely dismissive) and many had only a superficial awareness of *sardi-garmi* principles. Some considered themselves to adhere to the system but in practice this simply meant limiting intake of very hot or cold foods.

Among those with some awareness of *sardi-garmi* beliefs, meat and very sweet foods, such as dates, sugar and chocolate were generally regarded as 'hot', milk and rice as 'neutral' and vegetables and most fruits as 'cold', although there were anomalies, such as yellow melon. There were also regional differences in classification, for example, fish was considered to be hot in some areas and cold in others.

Mehri – In my city (Mosandan) people believe fish is hot but in his city (Kerman) they believe it's cold. They eat fish with hot things. They don't eat yoghurt with fish because they believe it's cold … but we do!(to cool it down).

Some women recognised that certain habits, instilled in childhood, may have originated through concern for *sardi-garmi* principles although they were now followed without understanding of the underlying rationale, for example the use of *nabat* (rock sugar) in tea. Others, while not adhering to the system themselves, nevertheless applied it to explain geographical variations in food intake.

> Safieh – I think, (in the) middle of my country, the hot area, people eat more watermelon than other places ... In Tabriz ... the people like the sweet (things) more than in other places. Maybe (because) this place is colder than other places in my country and therefore they like oily things and sweets. ... The best sweets and candy are (found) in Tabriz.

As in the Mexican system (Messer, 1981), many women only paid attention to the 'hot-cold' qualities of the diet if they considered themselves or any family member to be especially vulnerable, for example, due to sickness, age or physiological state (such as pregnancy or menstruation); at such times diet assumed even greater importance. For example, it was suggested that babies tend to be prone to coldness which can be counteracted with a small amount of *nabat*. In old age, body base also becomes 'colder' and individuals may become susceptible to cold illnesses.

> Zahra – ... (L)ike (my father is) cold and he doesn't eat much cold food, because he believes every time he eats more cold food, it hits him – affects his digestion and his digestion goes bad ... (H)e gets too much water in his mouth ... that's the way he finds out he's got coldness.

In Iranian, as in many other cultures, certain foods have been ascribed specific medicinal properties (Lock, 1980: 96; Pliskin, 1987: 141). The use of these remedies in sickness comprises a major part of popular Iranian medicine. Frequently, the foodstuffs assigned such medicinal qualities are marginal substances, falling 'betwixt and between' the categories of food and non-food, for example, herbs and spices are common medicinal ingredients (Lock, 1980: 96). In Iran, a range of dried flowers, seeds, leaves and berries are also used and are drunk (steeped in water) for a range of conditions such as digestive ailments, coughs, sore throats, fevers, nerves and fear (Pliskin, 1987: 141).

> Safieh – When I cook (mint) like tea, with *nabat,* I don't know why but it works on me when I have a stomache ache. I think mint is good and ... liquorice for stomach ache.
>
> Mehri – Sometimes if they catch a cold (or) stomach (ache), then (I use) *nabat* with tea ... We use some dried herbs from (a) special shop ... When we have coughs, we use (quince seeds) ... I don't believe it very much. I think when you catch (a) cold you have to go to the doctor. You can use (herbal medicines) because (they won't) damage anything but sometimes people just use them and don't go to (the) doctor. Especially with children

... (they) may have a problem in future because they don't kill all the microbes ... I saw a child in the hospital, they didn't take him to the doctor when he had a sore throat, so after a few months he had a rheumatic fever, so I'm very aware if my children ha(ve) a cold.

Although Western medicine is generally believed to be more powerful than traditional treatments, herbal concoctions are often thought to be more controllable and less likely to cause side-effects (Lock, 1980: 136; Pliskin, 1987: 142). In this study, most women used a number of herbal remedies, in particular mint water and *nabat*, for minor ailments. Such remedies might also be tried before resorting to pharmaceuticals, or they might be used as an adjunct to medical treatments, in order to offset their heating effects and restore the body to a state of equilibrium. In addition to the medicinal use of herbs, modification of dietary intake was widely reported by informants during sickness. Soups, fruit juice and plain foods were generally thought to be better tolerated and fries and spicy foods were avoided (whether these modifications were derived from Galenic-Islamic or more recent biomedical influences is difficult to ascertain).

Monir – If, for example, you get flu or a cold you don't eat spicy foods, you eat very plain foods, like just *kateh* – steamed rice, with yoghurt, or you eat soups ... watery soups – not too much spice in it.

A number of conditions required the therapeutic use of more commonly consumed foods, for example, honey, sugar and chocolate. For example, one informant described being prone to low blood pressure, particularly at the end of her menstrual cycle. Her account reveals the way she intuitively senses which foods to eat, on the basis of bodily sensations, and reveals her resistance to accept the biomedical diagnosis, in the light of her successful self-treatment.

Soraye – My blood pressure is a bit low ... I'm better off with the hot (foods) because when I eat too much cold food I feel dizzy. I start getting headaches ... Here it's more noticeable – I don't know why – because of weather ... here you feel (you need) to eat more chocolate but (not) in Iran. ...
I went to the doctor. They said they think it's migraine ... but I don't think so, because yesterday I had 3 glasses of milk with honey. Everytime I felt I was getting a headache I had one glass of milk and honey and it stopped.

In contrast to this informant, who had no formal biomedical training, another woman, trained as a midwife in Iran, applied her knowledge in a description of the use of *sardi-garmi* principles by couples wanting a child of a specific sex (hot foods are believed to encourage the development of a boy and cold ones to increase the chances of carrying a girl).

Safieh – ... My cousin used *sardi-garmi* for (the) sex of (her) baby. She wanted a girl and she can't get a girl ... and she said to me she used this (and it worked).

I think I believe some food could have (an) effect on (the) sex of (the) baby because it changes (the) pH of (the) body and (has an) effect on (the) move(ment) of sperm in (the) body of women.

Her explanation for the success of the method illustrates how traditional and modern concepts are syncretised and how the traditional may be reinterpreted and translated in terms of dominant ideologies such as biomedicine. She personally does not have confidence in the Galenic tradition, partly because she lacks the experiential physical evidence of its efficacy and in part owing to her training, yet, recognising the prevalence and persistence of this classificatory system, she offers a rationale for its success, couched in terms of the hegemonic medical discourse.

Safieh – I don't believe hot-cold but I think its connected to sympathetic and parasympathetic nerves ... for example yoghurt is *sard* and I think it works on ... the gland ... in our mouth and it makes water in our mouth ... because they say the *sardi* makes water in the mouth ... My mother-in-law believes you shouldn't eat fish and yoghurt together ... but I've never obeyed ... (the) present generation doesn't believe ... When I was a child somebody said don't eat yoghurt or *kaskh* (fermented yoghurt) with *ashe reshte* but I did and nothing happened.

I think ... in addition the energy of the food. Because the sweet and the chocolate is *garm*. The yoghurt is cold (less energy).

Nutrition and Health Discourses and the Differentiation of Identities

Safieh also considers herself, as a member of the younger generation, to be more enlightened than older people. This was a theme drawn out by most informants, not just with regard to dietary traditions but also in relation to other aspects of life style. In this study, the age of the women interviewed ranged from the midtwenties to the early fifties and the length of residence in the U.K. varied from two to ten years (some had also spent several years in other Western countries). All had been exposed to nutrition information in Iran and in Britain. Many interviewees regarded *sardi-garmi* to be based on superstition and considered it now to be outdated; generally younger women seemed to find the scientific 'facts' more persuasive.

Safieh – I hope I work good nutrition when I am cooking. For example, usually (when) I cook (iron-containing) food ... – (it) needs vitamin C – because I've heard it's absorbed better ... When I cook lentils, I add the lemon juice to it, or some tomato juice, because I know its better. And one of my teachers said the Iranian people eat onion with rice and kebab because there is glutamic acid in onion and (not) in rice and they complement each other.

Even among those most convinced of the value of *sardi-garmi* beliefs, they were not the dominant concern in ensuring a physiologically sound diet for the family. Rather, these principles were dynamically and variably integrated, or used in conjunction with popular understandings of biomedical nutrient classifications. Some foods, and in particular, fruit were widely perceived to be good for health – 'I think if a child has fruit enough ... she will be healthy (Goli). This was partly due to an awareness that they were considered 'healthy' by dietetic standards and they were preferred as a means of restoring balance to other alternatives. In some instances there was some ambivalence demonstrated towards foods which were valued for their heating qualities but were regarded as dangerous in terms of their nutritional value. This particularly applied to chocolate, which as James has argued, also occupies a structurally marginal position and is regarded with much ambivalence by British consumers (James, 1990).

> Soraye – I don't want to give her chocolate ... Dates are hot and better than chocolates, because eating too much chocolate can make you fat. ...

In contrast to the scepticism often acknowledged towards traditional wisdom, no informants expressed any disbelief of the nutrition information they had acquired. Like British Asian women in Scotland (Bradby, 1995) these interviewees used their nutrition knowledge to rationalise and to confirm the logic of systemic beliefs but unlike the Scottish group, they did not appear to reciprocally apply traditional principles to interrogate scientific 'reductionist' knowledge. In some cases informants used the nutrition discourse to assert regional superiority and in one case it also served as a means of expressing marital tension.

> Mehri – In (my husband's) city (they) eat too many sweets ... and dates ... they are hot because (they) are very sweet ... I can't eat. They make *fesenjun* very sweet but I don't like it. We have a problem with that, he likes really sweet and I don't like ... not very good for health, especially in his family ... most of his family they are diabetic ... and I'm afraid of it ... My family ... when they grow older, they are very careful with their food, they don't eat meat too much, especially lamb meat and not very fatty food. They use mainly vegetable food ... very good on sport everybody in our city.

Despite the privileging of the biomedical discourse over traditional knowledge, women commonly indicated that as their nutritional awareness had grown, so they had become increasingly convinced of the natural goodness and superiority of the Iranian diet. This was most strongly articulated by an informant who had spent half of her life abroad.

> Monir – ... In Iran they don't talk about foods the way they do here. It just comes naturally because all the diet,the Iranian diet is very good, when you think about it. (When) you get more information about healthy food. ... then you realise that what you had – the diet that you had in Iran – was healthy ... The people don't have any knowledge about what healthy food is, it comes naturally because it's been given to them, generation from generation.

The preparation of healthy food was considered to be an intuitive ability, born and bred into Iranian women. For those well versed in the professional discourse, such as one interviewee, who had recently completed a Master's course in Nutrition, this had provided reassurance as to the soundness of the Iranian diet and of the reliability of her instinctive knowledge.

> Hamideh – (Before) I didn't know much about it, but I just realised that, I think, it's so nutritious and ... var(ied) and you know, (the) combination of ... beans and meat and herbs. I feel, I realise, it's really worth it ... It's not just a lot of meat – you know, you just worried about cancer – too much fat ... The protein of plants is much more (healthy) ... I mean after the course I understand ... (and) I trust it.

If health information had generally shaped women's opinions, the nutrition message which had most powerfully influenced their day-to-day food preparation was a concern over dietary fat intake and this was reflected in a considerable degree of ambivalence regarding the taste of fat containing dishes. Although all informants without exception mentioned fat as a consideration, this was manifested in different ways. For those who had lived in the U.K. for relatively short periods (two or three years) the predominant focus was on avoiding heart disease.

> Mehri – I use a little bit of fat ... I don't fry the chicken or meat ... Some Iranian women, they used fat a lot, but not now ... Because the oil is expensive, you know, in Iran now, so they have to be careful ... Before – my grandfather's time – ... they ate fat a lot, because they work(ed) a lot ... so they used the fat, they spent a lot of calories ... but now people use cars all the time ... people use vaccuum cleaners or washing machines ... They don't work a lot, so they don't need a lot of calories, so they must be careful ... We have a programme on the TV to tell people to be careful. And when you see your friend has (a) heart attack and the reason is he or she (is) eating too much fat or a lot of sweets, you just wake up to yourself and be careful ... I use fish a lot, I don't know (if) it's true or not (but) I heard it's good to keep out the heart attack.

Her lay theorising interweaves an understanding of the biomedical discourse (i.e., the need to balance energy intake and expenditure), with observations of the influence of socioeconomic and lifestyle transformations, and she illustrates how personally relevant experience may prove to be a catalyst which transforms theoretical knowledge into behavioural change (Davison et al, 1991).

Among those who had lived in Britain for longer periods, concern with fat intake was more clearly articulated in relation to weight control. A number of women reported having put on weight here; this was often attributed to the need to eat more in a cold climate, and in some cases, to lack of exercise; three informants joined 'Weight-Watchers' during the course of this field work!

> Monir – We are quite conscious about (our) weight.
>
> We tend to choose less fat in our diet ... and we don't have any sauces, apart from salad cream and a little bit of olive oil and some fresh lemon juice but we tend to completely avoid sauces – mayonnaise and all that stuff.

Others reflected approvingly on the fact that they had initially lost weight when they came to Britain, due to the change in routine. From their accounts, it appears that the pressure to conform to western societal norms regarding body image may be experienced more intensely as the length of exposure to them increases. A significant difference between Iranian and British conceptions of ideal body size was remarked upon by some women.

> Soraye – (H)onestly, in (Iran) you just notice they are fat. I don't know (if) they wear something – (that makes them) look fatter. Yes, but when you compare it, (it's) not like here, I think they are much more comfortable in Iran.
>
> Zahra – (In Iran) people were not that fussy because, I think, they all wear these long veils, so they're not really bothered about weight, you know, having (a) big bum or big bust or anything like that, it's not showing ... I don't think people like it, you know, (being too) slim, you know, like size 8. They won't like that at all ... I think people prefer size 12, back home (and) they don't mind size 14–16. ...

It was also noted that weight loss was often met by resistance from family members (especially parents) in Iran. This was explained in terms of a generational change in ideals, with larger proportions, as an indication of a plentiful diet, being more highly valued among older people.

> Farah – I think sometimes older age women like people to be a bit fatty, rather than skinny ... I think because we think about being fashionable, maybe and they don't. That's why, when I married, my mother-in-law liked me being chubby ...
>
> Soraye – My father definitely didn't like. They think it doesn't suit you – being skinny, you're better being a bit (chubby). Last time I went to Iran, I don't know why that happened to me, for a week I couldn't eat ... I lost

weight ... I looked a bit tired ... but honestly I wasn't dieting ... They didn't like it, even my friends said, 'it's enough – eat something' (laughs) ... I don't mind it happening, I lose weight ...

Farah – I think when you lose weight, it affects your face and that's why they don't like. Really, I don't like as well ... You have lines and everything but your body is good, it looks nice but not your face and that's why they don't like.

Although these women discuss weight loss primarily in terms of aesthetic appearance, I suggest that additionally, for parents of Iranians living in Britain, the transformed body symbolises a change of identity, which in a culture where the harmony and stability of the family is so important, may give rise to a significant degree of sociocultural dissonance (see also Harbottle, 1995: 35). An alteration in facial characteristics is cause for particular concern, as the face is so prominent and is a focal area for inscribing identity, for example through hairstyle and makeup (Synnott, 1993: 120). This may be intensified in a society where the rest of the body is shrouded from public view, as in the Islamic Republic of Iran.

In this chapter I have illustrated how, as they go about the everyday business of feeding their families Iranian women deploy health discourses, not only to ensure the nutritional adequacy of the food consumed but also to assert their own identities (and those of their families) and to mark their difference from others. The relationship between food intake, identity-maintenance and health will be explored further in the following chapter.

6. INCORPORATION, IDENTITY AND HEALTH

The previous chapters have begun to consider the ways in which domestic food-work involves identity-work. This chapter continues that focus by exploring how Iranian settler women in Britain attempt to maintain the identities of themselves and their families as Iranian through their food-provisioning tasks. It examines how the ingestion of food may be a dangerous business, fraught with biological risks, such as poisoning, and associated culturally with a fear of pollution. The section then explores the dilemma of Iranian women, obliged to purchase foodstuffs which they perceive to contain toxins, such as pesticides and hormones, and how this may represent a deeper fear of being contaminated by western cultural values. Finally, it describes how women resolve their dilemma and applies a modified version of Lévi-Strauss's culinary triangle to demonstrate how, through their food-preparation rituals, skill and labour and by the application of specific cooking techniques and ingredients they are able to positively transform potentially dangerous raw ingredients into nourishing and satisfying cooked meals, and in the process obtain respect, power and status within their families and within the wider community.

West-toxification and Diet

Fischler has observed how the act of incorporation may be associated with deep-rooted anxiety:

> Clearly, the eater's life and health are at stake whenever the decision is taken to incorporate, but so too are his place in the universe, his essence, his nature, in short his identity. An object inadvisedly incorporated may contaminate him, insidiously transform him from within, possess him or rather depossess him of himself. (Fischler, 1988)

Neophobia in children and distrustful behaviour in adults may be observed when individuals find themselves exposed to new, unknown or suspicious foods. Physiological manifestations, including nausea and sweating may arise from what is essentially a socio-cultural taxonomic problem if, for example, an unknown food is suspected of being a taboo item. The serving of *haram* or impure foods to Muslims (including meat from animals not killed in the prescribed way and blessed in the name of Allah, pigs and blood from meat) may elicit just such a response.

In this study, the majority of people interviewed did not strictly adhere to the Muslim food code, but it retained a residual significance and their taste perceptions had obviously been moulded by their religious upbringing. Most avoided pork and ham completely, although they would occasionally buy frankfurters or other pork-containing products. Those who had eaten pork had seemingly developed a culturally conditioned aversion to it and observed that it had a 'dirty' taste which they disliked. Most saw no need to integrate it into their well-established and varied culinary repetoire.

Among those interviewed more general anxieties concerning food consumption also demonstrated a dimension specific to Iranian society. For example, during an interview with his wife in which we were discussing dietary fat intake, Mahmood interjected to describe the loss of traditional Iranian consumption patterns and their replacement with western dietary practices.

> Mahmood – Most of the Iranian foods are made of grains. Gradually during the Shah's time it became a mode ... to have more meat in food because they sa(id) those grainy foods are old-fashioned ... they don't have any protein ... (But) chickpeas ... are the best source of glutamic acid ... which is the kind of nutrient that neurons usually consume ... We not only have this in our ... main food ... but we also fry these and we mix them with raisins and we give (them) to children to take to school ... They say, 'take these things away, they're no good and go and have more meat. Look, westerners are eating more meat ... let's have more meat'!

Ironically, he employs the biomedical discourse to criticise the western diet and to lament the impact of the former Shah's modernisation programmes.

In Mahmood's account, there is a powerful resonance with the notion of *gharbzadegi* (west-toxification), a term applied in Iran to express the cultural intoxification of Iranian youth with western secular values and material goods (Farman Farmaian with Munker, 1992: 356-57; Sreberny-Mohammadi and Mohammadi 1994: 96-97). As I have illustrated in Figure 2, the medically harmful effects of the western diet, manifested by high levels of heart disease, are

Figure 2: Nutritional and moral valuations of foods.

Grains	↑ fibre	nutritionally
humble food	↓ fat	and
Iranian		morally sound
Meat	↑fat	↑ risk heart disease and
↑status		'diseases of affluence'
Western		morally unsound

also parallelled by the moral valuations of certain foods, which may be further understood to symbolise the socially and politically damaging effects of western culture upon Iranian society. For example, Mahmood draws a distinction between 'grains', including pulses, which he considers to be simple, nutritious and traditional foods, and meat which he associates with western influences and a concomitant decline in traditional values and practice. Although meat is a high status food, consumed by the affluent (and those who wish to emulate their western counterparts) it is also high in fat and as such is implicated in the aetiology of a number of diseases of affluence. Grains, on the other hand, are low in fat and high in fibre and are therefore nutritionally and morally superior.

Following the 1979 revolution, measures were taken by the Islamic government to eradicate all sources of western influence (this included the destruction of cinemas and consumer goods) in order to protect the Iranian people from 'west-toxification'. More recently medical campaigns have been mounted to combat the high prevalence of heart disease in Iran. At a symbolic level these campaigns may also be understood to represent the response of the authorities to the threat of (dietary) west-toxification and their attempts to minimise the damage they perceive to be caused by it.

Although in one sense Iranian migrants may be considered to have physically embraced the west, and to have been incorporated within it, nevertheless they demonstrate a high degree of ambivalence towards western standards and considerable resentment over the sustained political and economic interference, particularly of the British and Americans, in Iran's modern history (Zonis, 1991: 104-106; Farman Farmaian with Munker, 1992: 252-78). Interestingly, conversations about food and diet frequently seemed to precipitate the expression of anxieties regarding identity issues and political-economic and sociocultural concerns were inextricably interwoven with attention to the physiological properties of the diet.

At times these issues were deeply embedded within the narratives, but at other times they were more clearly expressed. For example, Mahmood interjected again, later in the same interview; this time he directly considered the impact of other cultures and cuisines, upon Iranian (and his own) identity.

> Mahmood – We have lost our identity ... we seem a sort of bewildered people. Some people think like that, they have lost their identity, they don't know where they are. We have been attacked by so many tribes and countries ... We have been influenced by so many cultures that it's got sort of mingled, amalgamated culture ... Adaptation always (causes) a lot of stress and pressure on the person ... We are very adaptable, very hospitable, very respectful to foreigners ... but (that isn't) necessarily good. ...

Other interviewees expressed concern regarding the potentially harmful aspects of the diet in exile. Although the wide variety of foods available in Britain was commented upon, nevertheless, many women considered the Iranian diet to be superior because of its 'naturalness', and experienced considerable anxiety over the pesticides, additives and other contaminants in the modern, British, highly processed diet.

> Mehri – I had a problem ... I feel the hair on my body is more than before ... I think myself it's – they put hormones in the meat, especially in the chicken ... maybe that's why. Or fruit and vegetables, because they take them (a) few times a year, so it won't be normal. I mean in our country we use one time from the trees or the land – one time or twice, not more than that ... My children's teeth are not very good here ... they (are) marked ... and the water actually is not very good here.

Although at one level, this angst may represent a broader and very modern mass manifestation of the fear of harmful incorporation (Fischler, 1988), at another level there is a particular political specificity of meaning in the Iranian context. The chemicals and pesticides referred to by this informant may not only be considered to be personally harmful, but in representing the 'other' of the dominant society, also symbolise pollution and transformation by an unhealthy social environment.

The fear of ingestion of hormones may signify other and perhaps more urgent dangers. Although these substances are not clearly defined in modern lay understanding, they have strong sexual connotations, for example hormone replacement therapy and the contraceptive pill (Fischler, 1988). Recently, in Britain, there has been controversy over the gradual decline in male sperm counts over the last decade. One explanatory hypothesis is that oestrogenic substances, migrating from food-packaging materials to ingested food, may be responsible. Hence men's bodies are under threat of contamination and demasculinisation by female substances.

In the preceding account, Mehri was distressed by apparently noticeable alterations to her own body, brought about by consumption of hormone-containing British foodstuffs. In her case, the concern relates to the development of male secondary sexual characteristics. In the light of other discussions with women regarding sexual matters (see also Harbottle, 1995: 23), I propose that underlying her explicit anxiety may be a more insidious and powerful fear of contamination by western sexual morality and specifically the threat of uncontrolled female (i.e., less differentiated from male) sexuality.

Positive Incorporation and Well'th Maintenance

Although a number of interviewees expressed concern over the potential loss of their Iranian identity, this fear being manifest most cogently in relation to their children's dual cultural heritage, as I will explore in Chapter 12, incorporation also offers the opportunity for the transfer and reinforcement of beneficial traits and desirable transformation, both of the individual body and of collectively valued characteristics (Fischler, 1988). In Islamic beliefs, for example, food laws comprise part of a system which assures the believer of spiritual health in this world, as well as the possibility of an afterlife (Tapper and Tapper, 1986). Foods are either permitted and lawful (*halal*) or forbidden (*haram*). The incorporation of *halal* foods, together with their symbolic valence of purity and cleanliness, is seen to be well'th-promoting, as was expressed by a number of interviewees

> Safieh – ... we don't obey exactly the same things but in my heart, I like (to) eat halal ... I don't like (pork).

> Fatimeh – We are not hard Muslims but sometimes I like (to) keep ... (our) traditions and something God says ...

Few ate only halal meat, although a number did prefer its taste, describing it as 'sweeter' (as well as considering it to be more healthy, whilst non-halal meat, like pork, was sometimes perceived to have a tainted flavour. For example, after discussing how one woman attempted to lower her family's dietary fat intake, I was intrigued to discover why she used shoulder of lamb, in preference to the leg – a leaner and more highly valued cut on the British market. Her husband interrupted, explaining the religious underpinnings to what has now evolved into a cultural preference; in Islam the shoulder is considered cleaner and tastier – 'it has less blood left in ... whereas in (the) leg there is more blood' and it is regarded as only semi-halal (Mahmood).

In the case of those families who adhered closely to Islamic dietary injunctions, the interweaving of the organoleptic and symbolic aspects of taste was more obvious.

> Mehri – ... When (they) cut the head off the sheep or chicken, the way Muslim people do it, all the blood comes out from the body, to make it clean – it's better. The meat is more delicious, it's very healthy, because if they keep the blood inside the body it's no good.

For those who would soon be returning to life in Iran, a major priority for women was to ensure that their families did not lose their Shi'ite faith; one woman was particularly diligent in ensuring her family's consumption of home-prepared, fresh, halal food. Even if her children requested pizza or burgers, she ensured their acceptability by making them herself:

> Mehri – I want to keep our diet, our food, because we won't live here forever, soon we will have to go back there and I don't want a lot of changes.
>   I don't use the ready meal, because my children doesn't like and I don't like. It's not our taste ... I make a burger myself because in the shop it's not halal meat, so we don't use it.
>   English children don't like the pizza we make ... I think they put tomato or mushroom or sausage ... and cheese on but I made with meat, because we can't use sausage ... With meat, tomato and green beans and cheese. I don't like (mozarella) because it doesn't taste (of) anything, just like glue – but I use cheddar cheese. I think the taste is better but it's not like (in the) shops.

By reworking the pizza recipe in this way, Mehri effectively transforms it into a distinctly Iranian Shi'ite product, and by so doing she ensures her childrens' retention of Muslim values, a subject which will be further considered in Chapter 12.

Recycling the Culinary Triangle

Women like Mehri thus hold a key role in maintaining the well'th of their families through engaging in their everyday household-provisioning tasks. This they achieve, not simply by selecting and acquiring specific ingredients but also by transforming them according to the application of specific culinary practices. By performing their food preparation tasks in this way they are able to diffuse the threat of negative incorporation and to ensure that the food they serve to their families will preserve ethnic and familial ties.

The cooking process and its significance in marking a cultural transformation of the raw ingredients was first considered by Lévi-Strauss, as was detailed in Chapter 2. Although his culinary tri-

angle (1966) in its elaborated form has been extensively criticised for
the apparently arbitrary binary distinctions applied and for its highly
formalised attention to the deep structures of the mind, nevertheless
the distinctions integral to the basic triangle provide a pertinent
means of analysing this data. I propose that the triangle can be effectively recycled, if reinterpreted and applied in terms of actual culinary practices, which are historically contingent and subject to
modification and contestation.

According to Lévi-Strauss, as human beings we face the paradox
that simultaneously we belong to, yet draw a distinction between
ourselves and the animal kingdom. One means by which we deal
with this paradox is in the arena of eating; across cultures humans
have developed culinary techniques in order to culturally transform
their foods. However, practices and products valued according to
one culinary system may be perceived to be threatening or suspicious within another cultural framework. Thus Iranian women who
believe the basic foodstuffs in Britain to be contaminated attempt to
address this specific threat of negative incorporation. The ways in
which they achieve this task may be understood by the following
reinterpretation of Lévi-Strauss's culinary triangle (Figure 3).

Example (a) above illustrates the basic elaboration expounded by
Lévi-Strauss, in which raw food is subjected to a simple nature-culture
transformation. In this case, which symbolically represents the perceptions of Iranian women concerning their own unmodified food
culture, the raw ingredients (grown in Iran) are generally regarded to
be 'natural' i.e., pure and unspoiled. The elaboration of the raw foodstuffs, by the application of Iranian recipes and cooking methods then

Figure 3. Recycling the culinary triangle

a) IRANIAN DIET	raw food (nature)——————————	*sophisticated cuisine*	cooked food ————(culture)
		additives *no cuisine*	
b) BRITISH DIET	raw food (nature)—————	spoiled food —(denatured)———	cooked food ——(toxic culture)
		additives *sophisticated cuisine*	
c) IRANIAN MIGRANT DIET	raw food (nature)—————	spoiled food —(denatured)——	cooked food —(restored culture)

results in the production of healthy, nurturing food, which ensures the positive incorporation of the eater into Iranian culture.

In the case of British food, represented in diagram (b), the raw ingredients, grown in an unhealthy environment and subject to contamination by the addition of pesticides, hormones and preservatives, are considered to have undergone an intermediary transformation, prior to cooking. This accords with Lévi-Strauss's description of a rotting process, but in this case the raw foodstuffs are perceived to have become marked as 'unnatural'. The consequent application of English cooking methods, considered by interviewees to be unelaborated and lacking in skill, results in a second indeterminate transformation, resulting in a cooked product which is of dubious nutritional value and may be understood to signify the threat of west-toxification.

The final element in this argument, as represented in diagram (c), is that Iranian women in Britain, when preparing food for the family, are equipped to work an alternate transformative process. Although they are obliged to use ingredients perceived to be spoiled or 'unnatural', I suggest that through their personal application of particular elements of their own highly elaborated cuisine, together with the use of specific medicinal and/or restorative agents, such as saffron, pistachios, *sumac* and dried limes, their food-provisioning performances facilitate and signify the reclamation of potentially dangerous food. Thus, they ensure that meals are not only edible, but also tasty, nutritious and sustaining.

These performances may be variably enacted by women, according to their different understandings of and needs to maintain the ethnic identities of themselves and their families and the range of alternate means available by which they may do so. For example, for Mehri, the need to use halal ingredients is paramount; for others, the skill and precision involved in the preparation of ingredients is more important. Additionally, there may be times of special need, such as during sickness or when under threat for any reason; then extra input of foods considered to have particularly beneficial effects, for their medicinal or symbolic value, may be required. Special meals and events such as *No Ruz* and *Moharram* may may then also be interpreted as providing a tonic to boost the symbolic immune system of the family and/or social group.

This chapter has particularly highlighted the ways in which Iranian women in Britain attempt to maintain a sense of culinary stability and familiarity. Nevertheless, in their daily routines they are often obliged to, and regularly engage in subtle dietary modifications, which they incorporate in largely imperceptible ways. Warde has similarly described an inclination within the British diet towards tradition, continuity and stability (1997: 57), and he has also observed a simultaneous and contradictory trend towards novelty and change. According to Warde, these paradoxical tendencies are inextricably intertwined in the modern mind, and in modern institutions (1997: 75). The tendency towards novelty and change is more fully considered in Chapter 12 in relation to the playful approach to food consumption observed among Iranian youth. The tension between these two forces, of change on the one hand, and of continuity on the other, is also explored in relation to short and long-term processes of identity-formation.

Food occupies a central position in the social lives of these Iranian settlers and daily concern with food and diet is apparently important, not only to prevent sickness but also to secure a state of optimal health, through the preservation of individual wellbeing, familial harmony, social relations and ethnic identity. In Britain, Iranian women attempt the daunting task of maintaining the well'th of their families in the face of what they perceive to be specific threats of negative incorporation. In response, they continually manipulate food consumption, so strengthening and equipping the family to withstand uncontrolled assimilation into the dominant culture, yet at the same time incorporating modifications in eating practices. In the process women obtain respect, power and status within their families and the wider community, as will be considered in Chapter 10. In contrast, those Iranian men employed in the catering industry find themselves engaged in a low status occupation, from which they derive little respect and which entails different threats to their sense of identity as I will explore in the following chapter.

7. FOOD FOR WEALTH
IRANIAN ENTREPRENEURS IN THE FAST-FOOD TRADE

In this chapter the focus shifts from the private to the public sphere, from female-defined activities to the predominantly male realm of Iranian settlers' commercially oriented food-work and from an analysis of food as sustenance to that of economic commodity. The number of ethnic minority employees engaged within the British catering trade has been observed to be disproportionately high. Commonly, such individuals have language difficulties and few formal qualifications, thus restricting their opportunities within the labour market. However, in the case of Iranian men, many of whom are highly educated, their participation in this relatively unskilled sphere of work requires further explanation. In this chapter the complex combination of socioeconomic and political forces influencing their occupational choices and the resultant emergence of an ethnic enclave economy are considered. In this respect, the Islamic revolution has been of paramount significance as an ongoing transformatory force in the lives of these settlers. A recurring and dominant theme in these accounts is of a perceived spoiling of national identity since the Islamic revolution, and it becomes evident that in their work with specific types of non-Iranian food, these migrants seek to disguise and to protect their ethnicity.

The Development of a Commercial Trade in Cooked Food

Ties of kinship and social obligation are integral to domestic food-provisioning but throughout history food has also been supplied and consumed within a cash economy. Farb and Armelagos suggest that the earliest restaurants probably existed during the

T'ang dynasty in China (1980:194). The breakdown of feudalism and the rapid pace of urbanisation in Europe and elsewhere may have contributed to the swift expansion of commercial food production (Beardsworth and Keil, 1997: 105). It has also been argued that the French revolution and the associated collapse of the aristocracy, which resulted in a greater availability of skilled professional cooks, was a major factor in the rise of the restaurant as a social institution (Mennell et al., 1992: 81–2). With the increasing popularity of restaurants, a number of chefs also achieved considerable public renown and status. The cookery books written by these individuals (for example, Escoffier) not only became known as classic texts and guides for training of the next generation of chefs but they also significantly impacted upon domestic menus and cookery styles (Mennell, 1985).

With regard to the growth in takeaway foods in Britain, the nineteenth century saw the rise of the fish and chip trade, one of the most popular and widespread street foods. According to a recent historical account, the combination of fish and chips (originally sold by separate vendors) had become an established institution throughout most of industrial England (with a particular stronghold in Lancashire) by the early 1900s (Walton, 1992: 25–26). Fish and chips rapidly became an important component of the diets of the working class, despite the prejudice and opposition to these foods demonstrated by nutrition and health professionals of the time.

The industrial revolution precipitated a wave of commercial food developments, including the introduction of the hamburger in the U.S.A. (Beardsworth and Keil, 1997: 110). In Britain the Second World War created a sudden need for publicly provided, ready-cooked meals. This led to the institution of British Restaurant and Factory Canteens by the government, in order that women should be freed from the constraints of family food-provisioning and able to participate fully in the industrial workforce. According to Baxter and Raw (1988: 62) by 1942 over 108 million meals per week were being consumed outside the home, over half of which were provided by private catering outlets. Subsequently, postwar economic expansion in Britain resulted in a burgeoning demand for readycooked meals within the workplace; simultaneously, eating out gained popularity as a recreational activity. Since then, the consumption of commercially produced meals has continued to increase across all sections of the population and in recent years the market share and range of takeaway foods has proliferated markedly (Caines, 1994).

Ethnic Minorities and the Food Industry

People from a number of different ethnic minority groups have entered the catering trade, in Britain and in other Western countries. Indeed Walton argues that fish and chips probably evolved from the commercial activities of Jewish migrants to the East End of London, who fried and sold leftovers from their fresh fish vending (1992: 1). In the process, these migrants have often contributed to a significant reshaping of local and national cuisines. However, this appears not to be the case with regard to Iranian migrants in England, despite their considerable involvement in this business.

A number of observers have documented the tendency of migrants to seek employment outside the formal economy and have pinpointed their disproportionate representation in the food trade (Watson, 1977: 193; Tze Ching, 1992: 10; Parker, 1994). In fact, such has been the scale of ethnic minority involvement in the industry that, by the mid-seventies, Watson was able to observe that the 'traditional British institution' of fish and chip shops had been almost completely taken over by rural Hong Kong migrants (especially in the Midlands and the Northwest). In part, the takeover stemmed from the willingness of these settlers to work longer hours, as well as their provision of a much wider menu selection than their competitors (Watson, 1977: 194).

However, in these studies it appears that the proprieters were frequently relatively uneducated and rarely spoke English, which meant they had severely limited job prospects within the wider British labour market. They were clearly distinguished from university graduates of similar origins, who obtained professional jobs and more readily interacted with their British counterparts (Watson, 1977: 195). In contrast, the majority of Iranians working in this business appear to be fluent in English and have been educated to at least 'GCSE' and 'A'-level standard in this country. Many also hold degrees. Their movement into the industry therefore requires more complex analysis.

Moreover, Chinese, Indians and others entering the takeaway food industry have significantly modified the range of foods available and have facilitated the transformation of British tastes. For example, the current popularity of curry is so great that a number of media accounts have remarked upon the fact, and one feature writer in *The Telegraph magazine* recently observed that it may now be considered 'almost as British as roast beef' (Fishlock, 1994: 25). The success of certain ethnic restaurants may also be partially attributed to the influences of these migrant entrepreneurs (Watson, 1977: 195; Pong, 1986: 5). However, in the case of Iranian fast-food vendors, no such impact is apparent.

Iranian Migrants and the British Labour Market

Considerable attention has been paid to the conceptualisation of ethnic minority economic activities (Tze Ching, 1992). The terms 'ethnic economy' (originating from middleman minorities literature) and 'ethnic enclave economy' (deriving from labour segmentation theories) are often used interchangeably to designate individual minority employment sectors that coexist with the mainstream economy (Light et al., 1994). It is not within the scope of this chapter to review the wider debate, but I have accepted the contention that 'ethnic enclaves', which require spatial clustering and tend to focus on employee income/exploitation, largely overlooking the self-employed, may be encompassed within the more general and wider term 'ethnic economy'. This concept appears more salient to the analysis of Iranian migrants' economic activities, the majority of whom are business owners (Light et al., 1994).

It is often assumed that ethnic economies are homogenous; in reality, sub-groups composed, for example of different religious affiliations, have been shown to network separately from each other and to demonstrate markedly different economic clustering patterns (Light, *et al.*, 1993). There are no official data available concerning Iranian economic activities in this country (like other Middle Eastern populations, they are categorised under the 'Asian'; ethnic grouping for such analysis – Thurman, personal communication, O.P.C.S.). However, in Los Angeles (the largest single centre of Iranian settlement in the U.S.A.) Iranian Jews are more likely to engage in the wholesale and retail sales of clothing and jewellery, Armenians in finance, real estate and insurance, Baha'is in durable goods manufacture and health and legal services and Shi'ites in the construction industry and durable goods manufacture (Light et al., 1993).

In Britain, research on other ethnic groups also indicates regional trends. For example, Manchester was historically the international commercial centre of the textile industry. Recent migrants from Pakistan have, like Jewish immigrants before them, chosen to enter an already well-established clothing trade, carving out a specific niche by supplying cheap clothing which is particularly popular with market traders (Werbner, 1990b). This study is specifically concerned with the economic activities of Shi'ite Iranians. Although interviewees had settled in different regions – i.e., the Northwest, Yorkshire and the Midlands – there was a high degree of consensus in their explanations of the causal factors resulting in an apparent clustering within the catering trade.

Naser – I know why they all went into takeaways. Most of them, they came to study ... and then they stopped getting money from (the) government, you know, they couldn't get any more grant(s) ... so they started working ... and one of the first guys who really started it all ... he started a pizza place ... started to employ these (Iranians). They all got hard (up) and had to work there ... They all learned the trade and realised it's no bother (and) everyone likes (pizza).

A combination of economic, social and political influences are implicated in the movement of Iranians into the food industry. In some respects they are similar to those experienced by other migrants, in particular the difficulty of finding jobs within the mainstream labour-market. In addition, the Iranian revolution and subsequent international sequelae have impacted profoundly upon the economic (and social) lives of these migrants.

Initial Movement into the Catering Trade

Prior to the Islamic revolution of 1979, there had been a constant movement of Iranian students to Britain and other Western countries. These were mainly young, single and relatively affluent males, the majority intending to return to Iran upon completion of their studies (Gilanshah, 1990). However, the flow of government and private funding ceased following the revolution, forcing overseas students to seek temporary work to support themselves. Their political status, as temporary residents and the need for flexible hours of work also contributed to their choice of the fast-food trade. Reza's story provides an example of the specific and immediate impact of these events. He arrived in Britain in 1976, then in his early twenties. Wanting to learn computing but restricted by Iranian government funding policy, he instead studied mathematics. As he observes:

Reza – (L)ater it wasn't really important what kind of a course you wanted to do – unfortunately – 1978 – we had (the) revolution, so everybody had a feeling for politics, you weren't much concerned with what you were studying or whether you actually studied or not ... (but) I wanted to carry on ... (however)it seemed of secondary importance.

Upon graduation in 1981, he had hoped to continue to higher degree level, but, unable to obtain funding from the new Islamic government in Iran, and hit by a massive increase in overseas students' fees in Britain, he was obliged to seek temporary employment. His student visa having expired, he lived, like a number of Iranians at that time, under a constant threat of deportation to what he believed to be a hostile home environment, where 'Western indoctrinated' graduates were reportedly being imprisoned. His uncertain political status also restricted his opportunities to work and influenced his decision to enter the food trade.

> Reza – At the time I started in '81, I mean, my visa was just about to run out and it was only a visa for studying, it wasn't permanent ... and didn't allow me to work, so it had to be cash in hand, and usually the easiest kind of job that you find in that situation is catering ... Even with English students, the ones who want extra cash ... they usually end up working in the pubs or restaurants – any kind of catering business ... I always hoped I'd do something, take on a job which had something more to do with what I studied. ...

Like many less well qualified immigrants, he resorted to the informal sector of the labour market. Initially he worked for a few hours a week, cash-in-hand, at an Indian restaurant. Later, he joined a number of his companions serving in a takeaway owned by an Iranian friend. 'I only went there when I had decided I wanted to go into the same business. I just went to pick up some ideas.' (Reza)

Having sought political asylum in 1983, the stress and uncertainty finally ended two years later when he heard that his application had been successful.

> Reza – (T)hen I knew: I can either start my own business ... I had already saved and had some money (to) carry on studying ... (but I decided) to make a business first and then go back – not knowing that once you dip your head into it, you can't get it out!

He formed a partnership with one of his friends and, having taken over an existing takeaway, they initially sold burgers and a few frozen pizzas. As they built up trade and became more experienced, they gradually expanded the menu by adding a range of kebabs. They also improved the quality of the food served, for example by making their own pizzas. Business, which had been slow to begin with, increased steadily.

Their experience seems to be typical of those who entered the trade in the early stages of its development. Prior to the mid-eighties, the demand for fast-food grew enormously and there were few outlets so that it became a highly lucrative proposition (Pong, 1986: 4). As a result, in addition to those who entered the catering industry as students or graduates, other Iranians with professional experience also began to drift into it at this time. Their influx was not due solely to the 'pull' of the trade, it was also influenced by the decline in the British national economy. Mehdi, for example, had held a job as an electronic engineer but the recession led to the British company he worked for going bankrupt. He helped out temporarily in his cousin's takeaway and then he and his English wife decided to start their own business.

The Emergence of a Distinct Ethnic Economy

In the aftermath of the Islamic revolution and the Iran-Iraq war, increasing numbers of more permanent exiles and refugees arrived in Western Europe and North America. Their origins were more heterogeneous in terms of age, marital status, social class, religion, ethnic background and prior western experience (Kamalkhani, 1991; Lipson, 1992).

By this stage, an increasing concentration of Iranians within the takeaway business was leading to the development of an ethnic economy, which served to attract others. For example, Amir was married with one young child when he came to the U.K. in 1989. He was a political refugee, following imprisonment under the Islamic regime. Members of his wife's family were already settled in the north of England and he spent the first three months living with them as he tried to adjust to the way of life here. For the next year and a half, he worked for his brother-in-law in his pizza takeaway, then for another fast-food venture, before setting up his own business in 1994. The involvement of other Iranians was influential in his decision-making and reassured him that it was a successful means of providing an income.

Within the developing ethnic economy, bonds of trust, loyalty and credit served to further attract coethnics. Amir, like Reza and many other Iranians interviewed, chose to establish a business partnership in the initial stages of his business development. Such joint ventures seem to offer a degree of security if one or both partners are inexperienced or if the premises are situated in an unfamiliar neighbourhood. Generally partners who were Iranian but also wellknown, trusted and from the same ethnic and religious background were preferred. For example, both Reza and his partner were Azeri (from the Turkish speaking area of Azerbyjan) and had known each other for a considerable length of time.

Kinship ties (and occasionally marital bonds, as in the case of Mehdi and Fiona) were also good grounds for such a lasting partnership. In some instances Turkish co-owners were chosen, particularly if the Iranian was Azeri; less commonly, agreements with members of other groups such as Pakistanis were mentioned (apparently there are a number of Iranian 'sleeping partners' in the presently booming Midlands Balti trade). Generally, as is indicated by studies of other minority groups (Watson, 1977: 192), the goal appears to be to move towards individual ownership and expansion. Often the capital investment required is obtained predominantly from personal savings and family resources and both Amir and Reza preferred to take the time to accrue personal savings and to rely on additional funding from family members in Iran, rather than to be heavily indebted to British banks. Within ethnic economies, credit arrangements are also important, particularly in the early stages of business development.

Not only was the autonomy and flexibility of self-employment considered to be preferable to working for someone else, many Iranians had been repelled by the discrimination they had encountered within the wider labour-market. In a number of other Iranian migrant communities, those obliged to rely on the mainstream economy have also been demonstrated to experience occupational and financial disadvantage, such that highly qualified individuals are often obliged to accept relatively unskilled and poorly paid jobs (Pliskin, 1987; Kamalkhani, 1991; Light et al., 1993). At times avoidance of overt racial harassment seems to provide an even stronger 'push' factor. Hence, the catering trade may particularly suit the needs of this and other ethnic minority groups by providing an 'unobtrusive niche on the fringe of the British economy', allowing interaction with the host culture as far as possible on their own terms (Watson, 1977: 194).

> Amir – You can't get a job here if you're black … for example we have 20 (Iranian owned) takeaways – 18 or 19 owners have got a qualification … I know someone else, (he's) got a job in a company. They gave him a hard time and he left his job and went to (a) takeaway.

It is predominantly Iranian men who have taken up work in the takeaway food business, but a small number of women, like Floreeda, are also involved. Her account clearly illustrates the impact of discriminatory practices on the movement of Iranians into the ethnic economy. Prior to the revolution she had been an accountant in a car manufacturing company in Iran, but she resigned in anticipation that female staff would be forced out of work by the Islamic junta, and applied for a visa to visit her brother in Britain. A year later (1985) she arrived and stayed with him for six months. She intended to acquire a British certificate in accountancy, but, meanwhile, her brother had opened a takeaway and she began to help out. She then realised that even with qualifications she would be unlikely to find a job in view of the discrimination she perceived towards immigrants. 'I think they prefer English people rather than foreigners, especially when they know you're from (the) Middle East, it's worse … ' (Floreeda).

Instead, she invested in her brother's business. Floreeda now owns a twenty-five percent of the shares and considers herself to work part-time, with an input of thirty-six hours weekly! This also allowed her to undertake further training as a beauty therapist. When she started college she became deeply disturbed by the attitudes and behaviour of many of the students (mainly young, white, working class women).

> Floreeda – (T)heir attitude towards foreigners is bad ... they usually look at foreigners like this (demonstrates look of distaste) ... they don't want to get close to them ... if there is someone else they won't work with (a) foreigner ... You feel awful ... They watch you ... I hate that.

Her exposure to such discrimination has made her more aware of racism within wider society and she has become increasingly concerned at the apparent upsurge in racial aggression in recent years.

> Floreeda – I know a girl, she's Iranian ... she got a note (through) her door, saying 'foreigner go home' ... I don't feel secure ... one day they (may) realise ... I'm the only foreigner in this road ... (and) set fire to my house or something – what can you do? It wasn't like that five years ago. I notice it more (now) ... especially in college ... sometimes when I come home I say: 'Oh my God, I don't want to go back to college again'.
>   That's why I'm glad I've got my own job, I don't need to work for them.

Clearly, Floreeda sees self-employment as a means of protection against discimination from employers and/or fellow work-mates. Nevertheless, even on their own territory, Iranian entrepreneurs, like the Chinese workers studied by Parker (1994), are always vulnerable to the possibility of racial abuse from customers and feel the need to remain vigilant at all times.

Consolidation and Diversification

Whereas in the early days of its development, the fast-food trade was highly lucrative, from the late eighties onwards market growth has declined slightly, whilst the number of outlets has proliferated. Competition has become increasingly fierce, with intense price discounting by the largest chains, resulting in a squeeze on profit margins for all involved (Caines, 1994).

The soaring number of outlets has led to geographical diversification, with would-be entrepreneurs now establishing businesses in more peripheral zones (Caines, 1994). Traders are also constrained by the consumer driven market, for example, needing to provide an increasingly diverse menu selection.

> Reza – All the time you need to be (working) to keep increased sales going. I mean, probably now is the time to do a new thing – possibly delivery. Usually, once you do something new you pick up some more sales, then after a while it goes a bit steady, then either you introduce

something new to improve it again or if you carry along the same line it tends to drop.

Economists optimistically forecast that, with everchanging consumer tastes and expanding leisure time, the market will not become saturated (Payne and Payne, 1993; Caines, 1994). Nevertheless, Reza's experience shows that to survive traders need to be highly innovative and adaptive. Even so, success for small businesses is not easily guaranteed. Having expanded their trade, Reza and his partner decided to purchase a second outlet in 1989. However a combination of factors, related to the situation of the premises, management difficulties and poor accounting, led to its failure to generate income and the partners eventually had to get rid of it, after making huge losses.

Baqer was even more unfortunate; he too had succeeeded in developing a successful business and decided to buy a second outlet. However, this required high level investment and the new business did not prosper sufficiently to support the interest payments on the loans he had taken out. He went into liquidation and now, in his fifties, he is endeavouring to start again, at a stage when it is acknowledged to be particularly difficult to cope with the long hours and heavy work which the catering business entails.

> Naser – Age wise I think it's affected them as well, (when) they were young they could do several shifts, late nights. They all got, now, so many other commitments, wife, kids, family – they're finding it difficult – they can't work like they used to, so I think that's why they're trying to move into different lines. …

Others have attempted to diversify into less strenuous occupations. For example, Yousef has recently opened a gift shop and if it proves profitable, he hopes to sell his takeaway business. In this study, only one interviewee had succeeded in moving out of the food business altogether. He went back to college and is now working as a dental technician. His view, in common with many others, was that the small traders who had entered the fast-food sector prior to the mid-eighties and were now well established would remain successful, but for recent entrants, the prospects are fairly bleak.

> Naser – I know a lot of people who have started just recently and they're not doing well at all … bankrupt … too many of them about now … too much competition – Manchester, Sheffield, up north – Newcastle – everywhere … Even other takeaways – there used to be only a few Chinese or fish and chips but getting too many. Some of them I know, they're all moving into different lines … (Others)are established okay but it's not like it was before – a few years ago you'd open a place and guarantee … making it.

For many the desire to diversify is countered by the limitations of previous experience and established networks. Hence, Reza, who feels he has lost the opportunity to further his education, perceives his choices to be restricted to some other role within the food trade. Increasingly, as is typical of other ethnic minority economies (Werbner, 1990b), businesses have expanded both vertically and horizontally. Larger, highly capitalised firms have emerged at the lower levels of supply, for example wholesaling, and in Newcastle-upon-Tyne one key Iranian company reportedly dominates the entire British doner kebab meat supply.

Hamid is a distributor for this wholesaler, as well as running his own businesses. He came to Britain only recently (1990) having been active in the import/export trade in Iran. Initially, he had attempted to sell Turkish machine-made carpets but although cheaper than Persian handmade rugs, these proved not to be a marketable commodity during the economic recession. Realising that the trade in foodstuffs was comparatively stable, Hamid started supplying frozen chips, taking on sole agency for a Dutch company in 1991. He then intended to open a food cash-and-carry, believing he could attract enough custom from both Iranian and Turkish fast-food and restaurant owners to ensure its success. However, he was offered a partnership in a burger chain owned by a North American settler and recognised this to be a more secure proposition; it has since proved highly successful. Hamid has continually diversified and expanded his interests; he still distributes doner kebab meat, as well as overseeing his import company. In addition to chips, he now also imports tomato paste, 'pizza cheese', pepperoni and a particular type of sausage made to the burger company's own specifications. He intends to become increasingly self-reliant in future, for example by establishing his own burger factory.

Iranian Invisibility within the Catering Trade

Ethnic entrepreneurs within the fast-od business have commonly modified takeaway menus in distinctive ways. In Germany, Turkish entrepreneurs have successfully created a market niche for doner kebab such that it has become symbolic of Turkish identity. Additionally, by applying English language names like 'McKebap', which evoke associations with powerful multinational food companies, they have also been able to manipulate the meanings of the kebab and, in the process, have to some extent transformed the stereotypes of Turkish migrants (Caglar, 1993). Seen in this context, it appears particularly striking that, despite their large-scale involvement in the British takeaway food trade, the Iranian impact has been negligible (by comparison with, for example, the marked influence of Chinese food in this country). This is in spite of the view expressed by many of the Iranians interviewed that the British lack a distinguishable or developed cuisine of their own.

> Mehdi – English people don't have a food culture as such, they eat any food so long as it is hot but they don't know anything about it.

> Floreeda – I've heard that most Iranians (in the U.S.A.) are dealing with cars or petrol stations … but here it's a cold country, food is (the)best thing … (and) English people haven't got different types of food … just fish and chips.

The few proprieters who had tried to market Persian dishes reported that the taste had been too subtle for the undiscerning British palate. In most takeaways a combination of burgers, kebabs and pizzas were sold; some specialised only in pizzas. These were thought to be popular chiefly because they provided a vehicle for the consumption of chilli sauce, with hot chilli pizza being a particular favourite of customers! Interestingly, kebabs, identified generically as an Iranian food by proprietors, were sold in the awareness that the general British public consider them to be of Turkish/Mediterranean origin (Mehdi).

Food is a powerful marker of ethnicity and to allow one's food to be rejected or treated with contempt is also to face possible self-humiliation. The takeaway counter, as Parker has noted in the case of Chinese settlers, may potentially serve as a site for such contempt and for racial antagonism

> The counter acts as a transactions post, where money is exchanged for a packaged version of Chinese ethnic difference. Each transaction between a Chinese catering employee and an English customer has the potential to draw on over a hundred years of culinary repetoires whereby Chinese culture and Chinese food in particular have been exoticised and reviled as alien and grotesque. (Parker, 1994)

Although Chinese food has gained tremendous popularity among the British public, customers often continue to hold negative views and to make derogatory comments about Chinese cuisine, for example, the notion that takeaway meals contain cat or dogmeat. Moreover, Parker argues that the popularity of Chinese food is dependent upon the acceptance by takeaway staff of a continuing relationship of service and subordination, mobilised and reinforced by each face-to-face interaction across the counter. In the case of Iranians, by the serving of non-Iranian food, these entrepreneurs are perhaps better able to protect, as well as to disguise, their ethnicity. Not only does the food served – ubiquitous, relatively bland and global – give no indication as to the ethnic affiliation of the owner, even the names of many of the takeaways act to further disguise their identities. Many such names conjure up Italian-American imagery, for example 'The Godfather', while others simply designate the fact that pizza or other food items are available. The only apparent exception is demonstrated, not by those serving food to the public, but by the backstage food suppliers; some of these select names which openly advertise their nationality, presumably to enlist the interests of Iranian customers from a range of ethnic and religious backgrounds.

Sometimes proprieters admitted the need to use dissimulation and pretence in order to protect their identities.

> Floreeda – (W)hen I'm working, I'm not telling them this place belongs to Iranians, I'm telling them I'm Italian or half Greek/half Italian something, because I'm scared one day they'll break everything … Before (the) revolution I've heard that (to be) Iranian was (considered) very good, because they thought we (were) really posh, lots of money (and) oil but after (the)revolution (it changed). I can't tell them when I'm working I'm Iranian … Once it happened … I was serving a customer – daytime – and he said … 'what nationality have you got?' … I said 'I'm half Greek' and then he said 'I've heard that, a friend of mine told me, that bloke in here is Iranian'. I said 'No … we are Greek, we are not Iranian in here'. That customer, he was with a tattoo and rough … he said, 'Good, good, you are not Iranian' … that's why I have to keep quiet!

Her account highlights a perceived transformation and spoiling of Iranian national identity since the revolution. It also demonstrates the fact that all ethnic minority groups are not equally subject to discrimination. This is underlined by research in the U.S.A. among both black and white undergraduates, which indicates that Iranians are considered the least desirable ethnic group with which to interact as friends, neighbours or in the workplace (Sparrow and Chretien, 1993). Other studies in the U.S.A. also suggest that they are the most shunned and misunderstood of all immigrant groups (Hoffman, 1990). Most of those interviewed felt that to admit to being Iranian was to play on negative public perceptions and stereotypes, particularly of Islamic fundamentalism, and therefore to incur hostile reactions. The response of many of these individuals was to attempt to disguise their ethnicity and to pass as more acceptable others, such as Italians, Greeks or Turks, such is the comparative familiarity of Greek, Italian and other European foods that these are no longer defined as 'ethnic', according to recent food industry reports (Miller, 1986).

Although it is relatively easy for entrepreneurs within the fast-food trade to disguise their identities in this way and to run relatively successful businesses, for Iranian restauranteurs the problems are considerably greater as I will consider in the next chapter. Moreover, the involvement of Iranian men in food-work, which accords them little public respect, together with their perceived need to deny their nationality has implications with regard to their gender status as will be explored in Chapters 9 and 10.

The preceding account has illustrated the multiple and intersecting factors which have led to the emergence and consolidation of a distinct Shi'ite Iranian ethnic economy, paradoxically based on non-Iranian takeaway foods. There are both material and symbolic reasons for the development of this fast-food based ethnic economy. Discrimination within the formal labour market and nationwide economic decline served as key 'push' factors propelling the movement of these migrants into the informal sector, whilst the autonomy and marginality of takeaways, as well as their huge profitmaking capacity, proved highly attractive. Although competition within the trade has since increased and arduous working conditions are a powerful disincentive, nevertheless the takeaway business still provides a feasible prospect in an increasingly gloomy economy.

The immediate political and economic impact of the Islamic revolution was clearly a major influence in precipitating the initial drift into this business. Moreover, the longterm fallout in terms of deteriorating Western perceptions of the Iranian people and their response to emergent stereotypes, in addition to their own internal problems of national identity have profoundly influenced the ways in which they have worked with food. In the light of their perceived stigmatisation, the attempts to disguise their ethnicity by passing as Greeks or Italians, and the unwillingness of Iranians in the takeaway business to serve Persian food, may be interpreted as a defence mechanism, avoiding self-exposure and the possibility of rejection through the medium of their cuisine.

8. THE RESTAURANT TRADE AND THE INVISIBILITY OF IRANIAN CUISINE

The popularity of ethnic foods in Britain has soared over the past twenty years or so. Italian, Indian and Chinese dishes have now become well-established favourites, such that, as I mentioned in the last chapter, curry now threatens to replace roast beef and yorkshire pudding as the national dish. Recently other food traditions, notably those of Thai, Mexican and Japanese origin have also made significant inroads in the ethnic food market. However, despite the aesthetic sophistication of Iranian cuisine, it has had little apparent impact within the British ethnic food sector and there are relatively few successful Iranian restaurants in this country. This chapter considers the factors which enable restaurant owners to enlist the interests of potential consumers and explores why Iranian entrepreneurs, who have proved highly successful in other ventures, have seemingly failed in this regard. Among other factors, the chapter illustrates how the despoiling of Iranian identity wrought by international responses to the Islamic revolution has proved a powerful deterrent to would-be restaurateurs.

Globalisation and the Diffusion of Cuisines

The late modern world is one in which individual nation states continue to engage in the construction of a national culture, of which cuisine is a key element; simultaneously such constructions are modified, contested and reinforced by both local and global influences (Zubaida, 1994a: 39–41). For example, a national cuisine may share a common set of flavour principles but these are subject to regional and local variation of expression (as described in Chapter 4). Throughout history, there has been a continual diffusion of influences across national boundaries within a particular geographical location. However, recently, processes of globalisation have had an increasing impact upon national cultures and cuisines. International tourism, migration, communication and trade links have all been important in this respect and have resulted in somewhat diverse effects. At times global processes have led to a movement towards homogenisation, for example with the proliferation of McDonalds outlets throughout the world. At other times the effect has been a resurgence of interest in local cuisines, perceived by the public to be in danger of extinction, as is currently the case with respect to some British regional traditions.

Tourism has proved to be a particularly powerful force in shaping food cultures. For example, it has resulted in 'the banalisation' of much of the food served at resorts catering to the tastes of package holidaymakers, with fish and chips and a variety of bland items appearing on the menus of restaurants and tavernas in various parts of the Mediterranean. On the other hand, recently there has been increasing demand from more affluent and discriminating tourists for exotic food and 'authentic' menus (Zubaida, 1994a: 44–45). Locally the response to this demand has precipitated a search for traditional (and often almost forgotten) dishes by international hoteliers, as well as by local entrepreneurs.

In the West, those who have travelled abroad continue to be influenced by their holiday exposure (sometimes in the short-term this may be linked with a nostalgic desire to recapture holiday memories) and increasingly seek out exotic cuisines at home. Entrepreneurs from migrant communities have responded to this search, with the resultant growth in the 'ethnic' food sector. However, despite the rapid growth in popularity of 'ethnic' restaurants generally (Miller, 1994: 19), there appear to be very few Iranian eating places in this country.

The Relative Failure of Iranian Restaurants in Britain

There may be a number of reasons, encompassing economic as well as social influences, which determine the success or failure of a restaurant. Firstly, such ventures require a much greater level of capital investment than do fast-food outlets. The level of financial risk, especially during the economic decline of the eighties was one factor which appears to have deterred would-be investors.

> Amir – After (the) recession Iranians didn't take a risk to open a restaurant because so many restaurants went bankrupt. That's why we stick with fast food.

> I could take a risk with Italian food – people in England know Italian food but they don't know Iranian food.

Nevertheless, despite the economic recession, the U.K. consumer catering market has expanded considerably over the last fifteen years (by 69 percent between 1986 and 1992); although this figure includes consumption of takeaway foods, the restaurant sector has also increased substantially (Payne and Payne, 1993). Public houses and hotels remain the most common eating venues but ethnic restaurants have become, and are forecast to continue to be increasingly popular. Economic influences alone are therefore clearly inadequate to explain the reticence of Iranian entrepreneurs to involve themselves in this sector of the market. Rather, it appears to have been the intersection of social and political with economic influences which has been crucial to the creation of a climate in which the British general public are not perceived to be receptive to Iranian culture or cuisine.

According to participants in this study, the Islamic revolution was particularly significant in this respect, first, in creating negative stereotypes about Iranians which were believed to deter the British from trying their food, and second, through the paralysis of tourism within Iran and the consequent lack of exposure of outsiders to that food culture. Some interviewees contrasted the unfamiliarity of Iranian food with the popularity of cuisines from wellknown tourist haunts such as Greece and Turkey:

> Fiona – If the revolution hadn't happened, Iran would have been a main holiday destination like Turkey now is.
>
> Mehdi – A lot of people haven't heard of Iran and there's Islamic prejudice. If I call it an Iranian restaurant, how many people am I going to get?
>
> Floreeda – I don't think a restaurant is good (here), especially Persian food, because (British people) don't know about Persian food.

Moreover, whereas other minorities, such as Pakistani and Chinese groups, have large and well-established local communities which continue to offer a considerable degree of patronage for their own restaurants, the Iranian population, especially in the Midlands and the North, is much smaller and more sparsely settled, rarely providing adequate support for a distinctively ethnic restaurant. Nevertheless, it was reported by informants in this study that there are a number of well-established and flourishing Iranian restaurants in Manchester and London. In these cities more concentrated Iranian settlements potentially provide a substantial market. Moreover, according to some Iranian interviewees, their relative success may be related to the fact that these cities are more cosmopolitan and the inhabitants may therefore be more open to new tastes.

Naser – I've had friends who started restaurants with Iranian food, some of them are doing OK, you know, it depends which area and what part, I mean some in Manchester (are) quite good … and there's some in London, quite a lot and they do quite well, I mean they even get customers apart from Iranians!

However, upon enquiry, the majority of such restaurants supposedly existing in Manchester appear to have gone out of business, although there is one which seems to be doing well. The whole family are involved in the running of this enterprise. They outlined other problems specific to Iranian would-be restauranteurs, one of which appears to be the lack of skilled chefs in Britain. This was partly attributed to the security of their occupational status in Iran.

Azam – (I)t is very difficult to run a Persian restaurant and you have to have a chef, a qualified chef and we don't have any. … (And the) food we buy – the meat is very, very expensive. And when we go to a Persian restaurant the main thing is (the) meat and it has to be good. …We have to pay a lot of money to buy fillet of lamb.

Like many others interviewed, Azam elects to apply the label 'Persian', with its connotations of former empire and preIslam, rather than using the more negatively perceived 'Iranian' identity. She stressed the high quality demanded in the preparation of Persian food and the precedence given to the place of meat within the meal, emphasising the fact that, unlike other food cultures, there could be no cheap alternatives. Nor could there be any simple shortcuts to the intensive preparation required, and she felt that the demanding nature of the job, in terms of time input and working conditions, was a powerful disincentive to entering the trade.

Azam – (I)t's very difficult – the person who cooks, like my husband; he spends most of his time in the kitchen. While he's cooking kebab, he's facing the big huge barbecue and it's very, very hot. You cannot stand it … most all of them are men.
(A)ll of us – 4 of us – we work really hard, we don't have any social life. My husband, sometimes he comes here and goes to (the) kitchen at 7am and doesn't leave until 10–11pm … this is our life.

Prior to migration to Britain in 1975, Azam's husband had owned a chain of kebab restaurants in Iran. Once settled in Manchester, Azam became increasingly bored with her domestic role and she and her husband decided to re-enter the catering trade together. They have now established a reputation among Iranians in the North and their current enterprise (designated a 'Persian-Mediterranean' restaurant, and opened in 1993) has attracted a loyal following, not only from the region but even drawing visitors from as far away as Scotland.

Azam – As soon as we opened, a lot of Iranians heard, and these were people who had been coming to our restaurants and following us whenever we opened a restaurant. Very nice people – classy people, I call them – very easy to work with. ...

(W)e never had (a) problem struggling, thanks to all our Iranian customers who (have) been following us and supporting us.

The Enrolment of Consumer Interests and the Transformation of Food Cultures

Business analysts are concerned to establish consumer attitudes and preferences in order to discover the factors which make for a successful restaurant. For example, Payne and Payne (1993) report the main considerations of customers (in descending order) to be quality of food, value for money, attentiveness of service, overall atmosphere, the welcoming of families, availability of parking, and convenience of location. Nevertheless, these general concerns do not explain why some types of restaurant are more popular than others and in particular why some ethnic restaurants are successful and others are not.

By contrast, sociological studies of McDonald's indicate that it enjoys worldwide success precisely because it has a theory concerning the interests of its customers and because it attempts to play upon their dreams and fantasies in order to increase sales (Law, 1984: 187). Hence, it 'stages its dramas' in ways that appear attractive to as many potential customers as possible: for example, in light of the current concern for a 'healthy' diet the nutrient composition of food items is advertised; in order to enroll the interests of children (and through them to reach their parents) a number of appealing activities, characters and toys are provided.

Similar analyses can be applied to explain the success of some ethnic restaurants in enlisting the interests of a specific sector of the population. For example, Thai cuisine has enjoyed a recent surge in popularity in Britain. Through observations and discussions with staff in a number of Thai restaurants it seems that several factors have contributed to their relative success. Increasing media coverage, and especially television programmes focusing on Thai cookery, and the impact of tourism and travel programmes have created a general receptivity towards this cuisine. Moreover, taste and aesthetic resonances with Chinese and Indian foods apparently attract people who are already familiar with local versions of those food cultures.

Furthermore, in one Thai restaurant, the manager reported that, apart from the high quality of the food, the aspect most positively lauded was the degree of deference demonstrated towards customers by the (largely female and exotically clad) staff. In this case, the enrolment of British interests may also involve a manipulation of customers' fantasies regarding power and sexuality and specifically of a subordinate and sexually available female other. Although few women may be employed in other ethnic restaurants, such as Pakistani and Chinese owned enterprises, a similar dynamic appears to operate between subservient waiters and white patrons. Thus, issues of race and sex, as well as class, are enacted and reinforced in the restaurant setting.

With regard to British perceptions of food quality, entrepreneurs from a number of ethnic groups have learned that in order to succeed in this market, some degree of adaptation of both menus and specific dishes (if not a total transformation) is often required (Tapper and Zubaida, 1994: 13). Throughout history, a number of 'invading' cuisines have been modified, and often changed beyond recognition, in response to local demand (Mars, 1983: 144). For example, the Chinese food consumed in Britain has been recorded as bearing little relation to any 'authentic' Chinese dishes (Pong, 1986: 5). Italian restaurants, too, may be more accurately described as 'English restaurants with an Italian style'. Here, long menus have tended to replace the smaller selection offered by restaurateurs in Italy. As Mars observes (1983: 144) some dishes, for example, spaghetti bolognaise, have transplanted successfully and recur on every Italian menu, others have failed to gain acceptance. Moreover, a number of dishes, although retaining the same name, have changed beyond all recognition. More commonly less drastic modifications, such as the introduction of thicker sauces has been implemented to satisfy British preferences (Mars, 1983: 145).

To date it appears that Iranian restaurateurs have been less successful than their counterparts in their attempts to establish a significant niche in the consumer market and so to enlist the interests of non-Iranian clients. This appears to be due in part to differences in Iranian and British food combinations, to aesthetic and textural preferences and to other direct, food-related factors, as well as to wider marketing strategies. For example, although Azam reflected positively on the success of her restaurant with Iranian clientele, she was aware of the greater challenge of suiting local tastes.

> Azam – I can say (the customers are) 95% Iranian … but we started advertising and people heard (about) it from their friends and they start(ed) coming.
>
> I wish we could get more students – hopefully we will, but right now the number of students is low.

At the same time, she displays some ambivalence towards the idea of attracting non-Iranian customers, perhaps fearing that their needs will clash with the requirements of the established Iranian patrons. For example, she describes their differing expectations with regard to special offers.

> Azam – What we call … special is different to what (British) people are used to. People think it's a three course meal, which it's not. We (are) selling two of the most popular dishes on the menu … a combination of fillet of lamb kebab and mince kebab and rice for £4.50 and the other (special) is whole spring chicken in pieces, flavoured in saffron … for £4.50 with rice … but I've experienced a couple of non-Iranian people (who) came here and … when I explained to them they were surprised (that) there is no starter and no sweet. …

Azam is aware that if her family intends to sell Persian cuisine to a British market, they will need to be prepared to make some adaptations. In particular, the discrepancy between British and Iranian preferences for sweets and puddings, which was explored in Chapter 3, has been problematic.

> Azam – We are going to advertise for students … We're planning to change the menu … and hopefully after that we can advertise (in) more places … I feel we have so many kebabs and rice and I find that a little dry for our non-Iranian customers, so we'd like to add (a) few more *khore-shes* – casseroles. …The sweets, I'm not very proud of the ones we serve … we're not the type of people who are interested in having dessert; you know, back at home we used to have melon and fruit.

During one visit to this restaurant, with an English friend, I also noted a discordance between my representation of Persian cuisine, based on home dining, and the meal served. To outsiders, the sight of the unadorned main dish, without the customary extras, such as *torchi* (pickle) and salad, appeared bare and uninspiring. When dining there with Iranians, I had, it appears, been able to apply symbolic value to the meal, but this aesthetic exercise was not possible with a non-initiand, and as a result, the previous ambience proved elusive on this occasion.

Nostalgic Reflections and Contemporary Cultural Fragmentation

Advertising and enrolment can only work if the message latches onto something which the consumer perceives to be desirable. Intrigued by the descriptions, provided by provincial interviewees, of a thriving Iranian restaurant trade in London, I visited Kensington, reportedly its centre in order to discover the secret of their relative success. Here, establishments were clearly owned by Iranians with different religious and political affiliations, as reflected in the names, decor and the dresscode adopted by staff and patrons. For example, some of these seemed to cater to the requirements of orthodox Muslim customers from a variety of nationalities. These and a number of Iranian-owned cafe bars, which did not serve food designated as Iranian, appeared to be enjoying considerable success. However, there were other Iranian restaurants which seemed to be less successful and even run down.

As Shelton has observed (1990) understanding the stage – encompassing the architecture, decor and habitus of the staff – can tell us a considerable amount about a restaurant and the kind of customer the proprieter hopes to attract. For example, the name of one restaurant I visited evoked images of a glorious Persian empire, whilst the premises themselves looked in need of a coat of paint. As in the case of other restaurants in this trendy up-market area of London, a minimum cover charge of ten pounds was set. Inside, the atmosphere was subdued and foisty, with a slight air of seediness. The lighting was dim, a worn carpet covered the floor and on the walls only a single freeze was identifiably Iranian; British light music played in the background. The waiter reported business to be slow and there were only six other diners during my visit – two Aquinas scholars, one Iranian couple and a British/Iranian couple (all were over forty years of age).

The chef informed me that he had been recruited in Iran twenty-five years ago to work in this restaurant. At that time it had been a thriving establishment, predominantly because of large number of Iranian tourists flooding into London (it seems that, contrary to the accounts I had been given, there have never been many British customers). Since the revolution, the number of Iranian travellers has declined and the business is now struggling. According to this chef, few Iranian owners have the marketing expertise to attract the British.

In the case of this and other Iranian restaurants I visited briefly, it seemed that the owners were not quite sure whose interests they were trying to enrol, or at which part of the market they were aiming. For example, a meal in this restaurant was not much cheaper than in a Lebanese enterprise resembling 'a grand European hotel on the colonial fringe' (Shelton, 1990) with its plate glass frontage, parlour palms, immaculately clad waiters and lyrical menu. Nor could it compete with some of the cheaper cafe bars, which successfully targeted young middle class employees, who wanted a 'healthy' and quick meal.

It seems that many of these proprieters are unclear about how they wish to construct and play upon British tastes. This may be due, in part, to the lack of an established restaurant culture in Iran, which according to Fragner (1994b: 66) dates back only as far as the early twentieth century. However, I propose that it is also related to the discrimination perceived by Iranian migrants to be directed towards them and to a postrevolutionary sense of spoiled identity, which leaves them unable to discern any positive interests within the ethnic majority upon which to draw.

Loss of a National Identity

During the reign of the late Shah, a clear movement towards defining a national identity, involving a 'persification' of the language (Tapper, 1989: 237), and glorification of preIslamic civilisation and empire, took place. This national construction was also shaped by the strong influence of western politics and culture in Iran, at that time. Although resisted by many Iranians, it proved attractive in the U.S.A. and Europe, leading to stereotypes of a sophisticated, intelligent and wealthy people. This notion of Persian culture is still represented within some circles and is reflected in recent culinary literature:

> (Iran) is a distant land, remote and mysterious; a land of ancient culture and often elegant ritual. It is also a land of remarkably good food ... many of its dishes can be traced back a thousand years ... When the Persians first conquered the ancient world ... not the least influence was the introduction of their food ... To (the Greeks), used to plain fare spiced with little more than hexameters, the sophisticated eating habits of the Persians proved fascinating and sometimes irresistable ... Even Herodotus ... commended the remarkable skills of the Persian bakers and cooks ... Indeed, the Persians thought the Greeks remained hungry much of the time because of the dreariness of their food. (Shaida, 1992: 2–3)

Cookery books are especially important in helping to create a national culture and cuisine, and, as Fragner notes, may 'tell us more about a peoples' collective imaginations, symbolic values, dreams and expectations than about actual culinary conditions' (1994b: 71). *The Legendary Cuisine of Persia* (written by an English woman married to an Iranian) illustrates the point. This book promotes a pre-Islamic national construction by evoking an authenticity and superiority of Persian cooking from ancient times and Shaida claims much of the Middle Eastern and Asian repertoire to be of Persian origin. The exoticised notions of culture and cuisine upon which she draws are appealing to European tastes, yet Iranians in the catering trade seem generally unwilling to adopt and extend these images.

Since the Islamic revolution there has been a major uprooting of former constructions of 'nation' and a metamorphosis of identity of

Iranians worldwide. For many this has resulted in confusion and a sense of loss, as was articulated by Mahmood in Chapter 6. Ironically, it is precisely those who sought refuge or exile away from the Khomeini administration who now find themselves most powerfully stigmatised by the current wave of Islamophobia.

Goffman (1968) first considered the stigma associated with certain marginal groups, including the disabled and some ethnic minorities. Murphy also observed the power of imposed stereotypes, fears and misunderstandings, and the constant battle of those who experience the despoilment of their identities to maintain a sense of self-worth by adopting defensive strategies such as social retreat (1987: 113–22). Dorman (1979) highlighted the specific role of the media in shaping international stereotypes subsequent to the Islamic revolution and its effects upon Iranians; his observations are echoed by participants in this study:

> Zahra – Probably that's the reason I feel I can't mix up with them (English) you know ... When you're talking about Iran ... they always say: 'Oh that horrible Khomeini and all this terrorism' ... but you can't – I can't, keep explaining (to) people what we're like. ...

There seems to be a significant level of internal confusion among exiles and refugees over how to reconstruct Iranian national identity, which appears to be reflected by the stasis apparent within parts of this restaurant sector. Accounts given by provincial Iranians of a thriving London scene, with Kensington at its heart, thus appear to be based more upon nostalgic memories which are somewhat dissonant with the more complex and fragmented picture I observed.

As Finkelstein has noted, when eating out we tend to select establishments where we feel confident that we will dine among others who share our values and we thereby mark our cultural boundaries (Finkelstein, 1989: 26–27). In the case of Iranian settlers in Britain, there is a considerable degree of mistrust between the many different ethnic, political and religious interest groups. For many Iranians the prospect of dining out, in the company of hostile or disapproving others, may provoke intense anxiety and discomfort. For restaurant owners, this raises the dilemma of whether to broadcast their own political and ethnic affiliations (as seems to be the pattern in London), or to endeavour to accommodate all interests (and to maximise their market potential), as has been attempted in Manchester.

The previous chapter explored why, despite the fact that Iranian-owned takeaways abound, few sell identifiably Iranian foods. This section has considered why there are so few successful Iranian restaurants in Britain. A number of practical considerations have clearly hindered the growth of a distinctly Iranian sector. Additionally, the ongoing reverberations, through space and time, of the Islamic revolution have continued to resound in the lives of exiled Iranians and the ensuing potent stigmatisation and cultural fragmentation which they experience are currently reflected by a sense of inertia within much of this restaurant sector.

9. PERFORMING GENDER
MEN, WOMEN AND FOOD

In Chapters 4–6, I explored how the performance of (predominantly female) domestic food-provisioning was important in maintaining the health and in reproducing and reinforcing the cultural identity of the family. By contrast, Chapter 7 illustrated how for (mainly male) Iranians employed in the fast-food trade, the performance of their roles more commonly involved the manipulation and disguise of ethnic and national identities. In the following sections I will focus in more depth on how food is used in the performance of gender identities. Individual foodstuffs may carry specific gender associations; food preparation is also gendered and within the domestic sphere is generally construed to be female work. In the next chapter I will examine how Iranian women's diverse and shifting identities are reflected through domestic food-provisioning. However, first I want to emphasise the interactional aspects of gender, as a process worked out between men and women in changing political-economic and socio-cultural contexts. This chapter redresses the balance common to many studies of food-work which rely primarily upon interviews with women; thus it focuses specifically on men's food-work in the home and the workplace. The section considers how for these migrants, the impact of religious, cultural and global influences upon notions of masculinity and femininity within Iran have been further entangled with other differences of class and culture within the diaspora, thereby creating considerable potential for the shift and translation of gender identities. These transformations may be reflected in the performance of their food-provisioning roles.

Jendered Rights to Food

A number of studies have indicated that cross-culturally, there are differences between the foods considered appropriate for men and women to eat. For example, red meat is more closely associated with men and masculine powers across many modern and traditional societies (O'Laughlin, 1974: 305, Charles and Kerr, 1988; Ekstrom, 1991: 145–56). Men also appear to have greater rights to consume alcohol crossculturally (Gefou-Madianou, 1992: 7) and are commonly thought to require larger portions of food (Lupton, 1996: 104). This seems to be associated with a perception of the male body as larger, stronger and more physically active than the female body, a view historically reinforced by nutrition guidelines. On the other hand, chicken and fish have been considered 'lighter', more feminine (and less sexualised foods) and women are more likely, especially in our society, to be vegetarian (Twigg, 1983). Sweet foods are also more closely associated with women, both literally in terms of greater consumption rates and symbolically, hence according to one wellknown nursery rhyme girls are 'made of sugar and spice and all things nice' (Cowan, 1991: 184; Lupton, 1996: 104). Additionally, women across cultures are often expected to practise 'maternal altruism' and to favour the needs of men and children above their own food requirements; Western women are also more likely to be on slimming diets and/or to develop eating disorders, than are men (Caplan, 1997: 11).

Although this subject did not comprise a key research question, nevertheless the data show that Iranian settlers in Britain hold similar views regarding gender distinct rights to specific foods; the association of meat and alcohol as highly valued and 'male' foods, for example, was very strong. In this case, what was perhaps more distinctive and noteworthy was the identification of *ashe* (soup/broth) as a female food with particular spiritual and health properties; the association offers a key to the interpretation of women's status within the home. *Ashe* in particular *ashe reshte,* is served on certain religious occasions, for example to mark the end of Ramadan. Additionally, if pilgrims go to Mecca, or if individuals are about to embark on a major journey, for example to visit family members abroad, women may hold, and preside over, special gatherings of friends, kin and neighbours, at which *ashe* is served and special prayers are offered for the traveller. *Ashe* is also commonly consumed by the sick, as a nourishing and easy to digest food and it is valued for its warming (thermal) properties in cold weather. At women's parties and *sofreh* gatherings, involving both devotional and social activities, *ashe* is commonly served (see Jamzadeh and Mills, 1986: 23–65 for a discussion of the importance of *sofreh* gatherings). Significantly, the properties of nourishment, healing and spirituality, attributed to the soup are also highly valued (female) skills, through which women attain status and respect within the social group, a point I will address in the following chapter.

Gender as an Interactive Process – Reclaiming Men

It has been commonplace in the sociology and anthropology of food, and in gender studies more widely, to equate gender with an analysis of women's roles, while the notion of man as a single oppositional category remains largely uncontested (Cornwall and Lindisfarne, 1994: 1; Peletz, 1995: 79). This is particularly pronounced in the case of the Middle East, for example, a literature search for this chapter traced 36 articles dealing with the position of Iranian women and none which explicitly explored men's roles. Current publications, for example 'Gendering the Middle East', also continue to be predominantly written by women, about women and mainly for women (Kandiyoti, 1996).

However, gender for Iranian settlers in Britain, as for other men and women, is not simply about individual performances but involves interactional processes, which need to be considered according to specific historic, political and economic forces (Ong and Peletz, 1995: 5). In relation to this study, it is important to consider how men and women interact within the domestic arena in the construction of their mutual gender roles. Furthermore, the substantial involvement of Iranian men in the fast-food industry also raises questions regarding the ways in which their gender roles may be enacted through the public medium of food-work.

Domestic Food-work and the Gendered Division of Labour

Gender roles are enacted not only by what and how much is consumed by individuals, but, of more central concern to this study, they are performed through food-related work. According to Fürst, 'cooking as the female contribution to the everyday reproduction of man seems to be a crosscultural fact' (1991: 119). A considerable amount of research has engaged with the gendered preparation of meals. Most of these studies have focused on western populations – Britain, Australia and the United States, in particular and have generally relied upon data from women. They indicate that domestic food-work is predominantly construed to be women's work and that even in the few households where men regularly undertake some domestic responsibilities, it is unusual for food preparation to be included (Coxon, 1983: 173; Murcott, 1983; Charles and Kerr, 1988: 50; DeVault, 1991: 99; Mennell et al., 1992:96–7; Warde and Hetherington, 1994; Lupton, 1996: 39).

However, a recent Swedish study suggests that although the overall pattern is similar there, apparently a greater degree of male participation in food-related domestic tasks exists. In particular, men are more regularly involved in cooking the main meal of the day and in the purchasing of food items (Jansson, 1995). According to Jansson, this is related to cultural differences in the perceptions of normative behaviour, i.e., although Swedish women do have ideal notions of the capable and efficient housewife, they do not, as in other cases (such as Charles and Kerr's British study, 1988: 50) consider it unnatural for men to cook or feel their involvement to be an unexpected 'bonus'. Rather, men are expected, and themselves expect, to take part in all aspects of housework, although not necessarily to the same extent as women (Jansson, 1995). Jansson also points out that in Sweden the decisions made regarding menu choices are generally arrived at by consensus, rather than by women deferring to men's preferences, as is commonly the case for Britain (Charles and Kerr, 1988: 69) and the U.S.A. (DeVault, 1991).

Jansson argues that the less marked segregation of gender roles in Sweden, particularly in terms of the right of men to demand and the obligation of women to serve may be crucial in this regard. He also asserts that it may be the operation of a patriarchal order, rather than the segregation of gender roles *per se*, which ensures the privileging of male influence over food choice within the household. However, data from this study contest his view; although Iranian society is a patriarchal one, nevertheless, women in this study tended to practise a consensus approach towards menu-planning, not unlike that described for Swedish society.

Additionally, and in view of the public/private distinctions operating in the Middle East and other segregated Muslim societies in which it is the men, not women, who routinely engage in shopping excursions, it is not surprising that many of the Iranian men in this study continued to do so in Britain. A number of them also cooked main meals at home, apparently on a more regular basis than has been recorded among British and American men, and perhaps more akin to the pattern described by Jansson (although with such small numbers it is only possible to make tentative parallels). Although the evidence was sometimes equivocal and contradictory, it seemed to be ideologically accepted by the majority of Iranian families that whoever was best equipped to get the job done should do so; although this is usually women, men do not compromise their masculinity by undertaking these tasks.

> Farhad – Man and wife just naturally work together as a partnership, like running a small business ... together they can do a better job than one of them on their own.

> Goli – My husband helps ... he does most of the cooking ... He's very interested ... and very good at cooking.

A number of men had learned to cook simply by observing their mothers or fathers in the kitchen. For others, the experience of living alone as students in Britain had been an important one in forcing them to experiment in the kitchen and in giving them confidence, although this did not always have lasting significance. Some men, like their British counterparts, catered only for special occasions (for example, making kebabs for parties and picnics) but those who particularly enjoyed cooking, were more proficient than their wives or had more time available also engaged in everyday food production. For example, for the duration of her Masters' course one woman's husband carried out the majority of the everyday family feeding tasks. Another man – Hafiz – also undertook the daily responsibility for ensuring that his children were fed properly when they came home from school, but in this case for slightly different reasons. His wife is English and is not particularly interested in cooking. Nor is she as skilled in the preparation of Iranian dishes as her husband; moreover, she is engaged in full-time paid employment.

Nevertheless, dominant notions of what it means to be a man or woman in Iranian society have been strongly influenced by their strictly enforced segregation within private and public spheres. Historically, relatively few women (although this has been variable according to class, education and government policies) have worked in the public sphere, the majority have remained at home and have retained control over that arena (Ghvamshahidi, 1995). In Britain, it seems that women may themselves be reluctant to give up the identities, power and status that their food-work affords them, as the following chapter will reveal. Hence, although domestic cooking is apparently slightly more common among these Iranian men than their British counterparts, the managerial responsibility for this work continues to lie predominantly with women. In families in which there are fulltime housewives with no other significant means of obtaining identity or influence, men rarely enter the kitchen. Women engaged in paid employment outside the home generally negotiated with their partners over the division of household tasks, some also encouraged sons as well as daughters to take cookery lessons at school, but they continued to control the right of access to the kitchen. In fact, two teenagers complained that they were not able to practise their newly acquired cooking skills because their mothers did not allow them to 'mess up' their kitchens.

However, because men also recognised the well'th connotations of food-provisioning, if their wives were not skilled or interested cooks they took over the responsibility. This was particularly note-worthy in the case of Hafiz (mentioned above). It was of major importance to him that his children ate properly, and he regularly cooked the main meal of the day (comprising Iranian dishes). This in no way undermined his sense of masculinity; on the contrary, it rein-forced his identity as a competent parent, thus demonstrating his maturity as a man.

The Relative Flexibility of Iranian Masculinities

Psychoanalytic approaches to male socialisation have tended to be based on Western normative values in which a process of individua-tion and emotional repression is expected. According to this analy-sis, the construction of male identity may be very fragile and in need of constant reinforcement (Fürst, 1991: 127). It is seen to require a severe separation from the mother and thereafter a continuous denial of femininity. Women's work may thus be seen as a threat to male identity, in which case men may shun activities so associated, such as the everyday preparation of meals. Indeed, there are some societies, like the Mbum, in which cooking pots may carry such potent female connotations that if men use them (other than in a rit-ual context) they are considered to be transvestites (Fürst, 1991: 120).

Sociologists and anthropologists have criticised such theories for implying that there is a single normative process of male gendering, thus overlooking variability within Western constructs (Messner and Sabo, 1990: 12; Cornwall and Lindisfarne, 1994: 2). Additionally, psychoanalytic theory, which privileges early childhood experience, fails to take account of other crosscultural masculine variants in which emotional expression and interdependence may be valued (Margold, 1995: 279). Thus, although stereotypical views of Muslim men reflect notions of rigid patriarchal discourses, some observers suggest that 'in fact Islam has long allowed a kind of flexibility and precariousness in the construction of masculinity' (Ong and Peletz, 1995: 10). By contrast, a number of men in this study commented on the defensiveness and apparent inability of many British men to sustain same sex intimacy (as has also been observed by Kupers, 1993: 45–46), and spoke of the homophobic responses they elicited through their own relaxed and close relationships with other Iranian men.

> Farhad – Here from the day you're born they even separate the colours for you. I mean you can't put pink clothes on your son. But what's wrong with that, I mean, what's the problem ... They're so scared of boys behaving like girls ... really scared in this country. Not so much (in Iran) ... I remember when I first came to this country, we didn't know they were so scared of it, and people ... (saw) us (lads) sleeping in the same bed or ... same room, you know cuddling each other or kissing or anything like that ... they just think 'oh that's it you must be gay' ... So I think, really, here the society is so scared of it, even though, I mean it's supposed to be okay to be gay ... They're really scared. They try to push the boy to be so masculine just in case ... We don't think things like that can change what you really are.

Clearly, same sex intimacy is not viewed to be threatening to gender status. Neither is involvement in domestic foodwork and as Farhad indicates, this appears to be due to the greater weight ascribed to biological differences within dominant Iranian gender discourses in comparison to hegemonic British male constructs. Accordingly, social roles and individual behaviour seem to carry relatively less weight in the performance of male and female identities. This reinforces the anthropological argument that:

> (w)hat gender is, what men and women are, what sort of relations do or should obtain between them – all of these notions do not simply reflect or elaborate upon biological 'givens,' but are largely products of social and cultural processes. The very emphasis on the biological factor **within** different cultural traditions is variable; some cultures claim that male-female differences are almost entirely biologically grounded, whereas others give biological differences, or supposed biological differences, very little emphasis. (Ortner and Whitehead, 1989: 1; original emphasis)

Nevertheless, appropriate behaviour and role play were not irrelevant. In this study, key male relational roles, in particular that of father (but also of husband and brother) were important in the enactment of masculinity, intersecting with and informing other meanings of men's relational and positional roles. There has been a tendency in gender studies to uncritically adopt a relational-positional dichotomy, whereby women are defined in terms of their relations with (predominantly male) significant others, such as fathers or brothers, whilst men are defined structurally, in terms of their roles as income-generators, hunters or protectors (Peletz, 1995: 103).

These data support those who contest the relevance of such an analytic approach.

> Hamideh – I think, men they care for the children very much ... I know a lot of families, things related to the children, like bathing, usually men do.

For these Iranians, quality family time was precious; tasks involving the children, such as helping them with homework or playing with them, were considered more important (by men and women alike) than was assistance with other household tasks. Being with the children was also necessary for the work of instilling Iranian values, which women felt they could not effectively do alone. Where fathers worked long unsociable hours in the fast-food business, the ensuing lack of time available to spend with the children was seen as problematic by parents. If the relative parenting skills of Iranian and English women was a strong point of contrast and distinction, this was equally the case for men. Whereas Iranian fathers were expected to prioritise time with their children, their British counterparts were considered to neglect their families and put their personal interests first.

In addition to their direct childcare responsibilities, as parents and husbands Iranian men are required to provide materially for their families. Crossculturally, an inability to provide such financial support tends to result in the depiction of lower class and unemployed men as relatively deficient in their masculinity (Ong and Peletz, 1995: 10). In this study, one (highly qualified and experienced) older man had been unemployed for several years. He appeared depressed and his unwillingness to help his wife (who was employed full-time in a factory) with household tasks appeared to have been partly related to the transfer of power within the household (as well as to his own loss of identity as a successful academic male). Not only had she taken over his role (and status) as the breadwinner, but she had also retained control over the kitchen management; his reticence to act as junior assistant may also have demonstrated a resistance to further imbalance within their relationship.

As described in Chapter 7, a large proportion of men in this study were employed in the fast-food business. In Britain (as in other European countries and in the U.S.A.) this is generally considered to be low status work, and it is shunned by most adult men; it is commonly undertaken by women, young people and migrants, often on a part-time basis (Leidner, 1993: 182). One of the most important factors determining the status of a particular occupation is its gender association. Workplaces are gendered both by the cultural interpretations given to specific types of work as well as by the gender of its occupants. In Britain and the U.S.A. tasks such as serving in takeaways, which require emotional labour and the display of positive affect, are primarily performed by women. According to McElinney men tend instead to perform work which is relatively affectlessness, for example in business organisations, or which involve the display of negative affect, such as in the police force (1994: 163). Leidner's observations of McDonalds outlets in the U.S.A. also suggest that hegemonic notions of masculinity construct American men to be 'naturally' more explosive and less able to deflect verbally abusive behaviour than women. Leidner argues accordingly that the demands of management that counter staff should be polite to customers at all times may be problematic for men who are not used to having to cover up underlying emotions such as anger and aggression (1993: 204).

However, in Iran, where female visibility within the public sphere is lower, men engage in a much wider range of work activities, including working in shops, bazaars, restaurants and other service areas. Furthermore, sociocultural constructions of appropriate emotional display vary greatly crossculturally (Pliskin, 1987: 44–78). In this case, not only does the work itself demand a show of courteous behaviour, but social norms in Iran also require polite, self-controlled, sensitive and respectful treatment of others; the public display of negative affect, such as anger or aggression, is inappropriate for men as well as for women (Pliskin, 1987: 72). Thus, for Iranian men in the British fast-food trade, being pleasant and courteous to customers, even those who become rude or hostile, may cause less of a disjunction with their normative expectations of male behaviour. In their accounts, these men employed descriptions which clearly defined their work as male, rather than gender-neutral or women's work, by emphasising its heavy, dirty, tiring and, at times, unsafe aspects, especially late at night. Few Iranian women were to be found in these establishments; those who did work in the trade were usually wives and daughters, who 'helped out' if finances were tight, and in one case an unmarried woman entered into partnership with her brother (as was detailed in Chapter 7).

Nevertheless, in Iran, working in a takeaway is also considered to be demeaning. Most of these men came from middle class backgrounds and many held academic qualifications or had professional training. They would not ideally have selected such an occupation in other circumstances. However, as settlers in Britain, these men were generally resigned to the fact that the economic decline of the eighties, combined with the impact of racism imposed significant structural limitations upon their occupational advancement. Thus for them, as Margold has observed elsewhere, the process of international migration and the impact of changing geographical, political and economic realities may result in a transfiguration of masculine identities and roles (Margold, 1995: 276–77). In the case of these male Iranian settlers in Britain, by their engagement in work on the fringes of the British labour market, and which is perceived by the general public to be of low status (and, moreover, associated with women), they simultaneously reinforce their social and cultural marginality and the subordination of their status as men.

The data from this study, although exploratory, suggest that Iranian men in Britain take a more active role in domestic food tasks than their Anglo-Saxon counterparts. Although the evidence is at times equivocal and contradictory, ideological acceptance of male involvement in this sphere appears to be associated with differences in the cultural valuation of biological, relative to behavioural aspects of gender processes. These Iranian men seemed to accord greater significance to the biological 'givens' marking sexual identity and they therefore experience less pressure to behave in rigidly demarcated 'male' behaviour. Moreover, domestic food-work is highly valued by Iranians, regardless of its gender connotations, thus it is not demeaning for these men to engage in such tasks. As I have previously argued, gender must be considered as an interactive process, between men and women, in varying social contexts. The migration process may have different consequences for men and women, and I will consider in the following chapter how in contrast to the downward mobility of their male partners, the respect and high status held by Iranian women for their traditional domestic food-provisioning responsibilities may be perceived to be relatively enhanced.

10. WOMEN, FOOD AND POWER

Food-work is generally construed to be female work and women's responsibility for the domestic arena, including cooking, has often been linked with arguments concerning their relative subordination. Moreover, in the case of Muslim women, research in the fields of medicine and the social sciences (and even gender studies) has often been influenced by Orientalist discourses, which tend to construct Middle Eastern females to be passive and subjugated and their male counterparts to be uncivilised and ignorant, their masculinity relying upon a domination of their womenfolk. However, as the previous section has demonstrated, there may actually exist a considerable degree of flexibility in Iranian Shi'ite male (and female) roles. This chapter explores in more depth women's performance of gender through their food preparation tasks and shows that feeding may in fact provide a major source of power for these Iranian women.

Performing Female Gender through Food-work

Cross-culturally, naturalistic views of the body exert a major, although variable influence over the ways in which individuals perceive their roles and identities (Shilling, 1993: 41). In Iran, dominant legal discourses construct gender as created by God and depict it as biological, rigid and absolute. Men and women are seen to have different and complementary qualities which cause them, naturally and morally, to be suited to different domains and activities (Torab, 1996). Individuals interpret and construct their gendered identity as a process, according to normative values and through interpersonal relationships and daily activities.

The acceptance of innate, biological differences between men and women (which are believed to be expressed through the personality, emotions and skills) was widespread in this study, as the last chapter illustrated. So too were associated notions of complementary gender roles – 'it doesn't mean we (women) are any less, it's just that we are different' (Hamideh). Iranian women are assumed to possess 'natural' abilities to perform food-related tasks, as indeed are American women according to DeVault's recent study (1991: 57). Indeed food preparation skills are considered to be highly important in the enactment of the female role, to the extent that some interviewees felt that women who lacked the ability were deficient in their female identity.

> Safieh – Sometimes they think (a) woman is not complete (if she can't cook) ... because in my country every woman should know about the cookery, (whether) she works or not, she must know. ...

Nevertheless, in practice, these received values were frequently contested or contradicted (as inferred by the level of male involvement in cooking and related tasks). Many interviewees stressed the importance of both familial influence and individual propensity. It was also acknowledged that some men inherit or develop the skills and inclination to cook, whilst some women do not. However, there was a difference in the perception of those skills, thus if men demonstrated competency in the kitchen they were considered to be particularly gifted. They tended to be more highly lauded for their efforts than were women who were generally expected to be able to cook well.

For most women, discussion of food inevitably led to talk about being women, mothers and wives. Food-related tasks were generally considered by participants in this study to comprise the most important housework activities and meal preparation seemingly serves as one of the principal means of self-definition for Iranian women. As was considered in earlier chapters, domestic foodwork is important in that it maintains the well'th of the family. Nutritionally it satisfies individuals' physiological requirements, whilst through their responsibility for cooking meals and bringing family members together to eat women ensure the cohesion and integrity of the family unit. This involves emotional as well as manual effort and may bring a sense of fulfilment and pride, as well as respect and status. Through preparing and serving meals women are thus able to affirm their connections and to strengthen relationships with members of their families.

> Leila – ... First of all you can enjoy (being) together and you can talk about different things and you can make a more warm family ... not just for eating ... but if you cook something for your family ... you care about them. You want to look after them and make them happy. ...

Although most of the participants in this study no longer considered themselves to be strict Muslims, nevertheless they observed specific aspects of the faith (as mentioned in earlier chapters). As with the

Jewish women studied by Sered, these women retained and enacted their spiritualities by the correct feeding of others (Sered, 1988). Shi'ite female identity is reconstructed by them, to varying degrees, through everyday food preparation but also through occasional religious observances, such as *Moharram*. The holding of a *sofreh* gathering (as mentioned earlier), which incorporates the vital elements of prayer and food consumption, is a key means by which women may attain spiritual power within the family and the community (Jamzadeh and Mills, 1986). Women are also responsible for the transmission of cultural ideals within their families and by preparing Iranian dishes at meal times, and festive foods for *No Ruz* and other culturally important events, they express and strengthen social ties within the migrant community. This may also be a means of commanding respect and status, as I will discuss later in this chapter.

Shifting Identities: Variable Performances of Gender

Life stage has an important effect on the construction of female identity, roles and status (Brown and Kerns, 1985) which may be reflected in relation to food-provisioning. For example, in Iran it was common, traditionally, for adult offspring to continue to live with their parents. Older women thus retained the power to control the food resources and feeding schedules of the extended family, thereby also ensuring their loyalty and obedience. In this way women were able to accrue greater power and authority over the lifecourse, relative to their male partners. This is illustrated by a well-known maxim which was related to me by an interviewee, i.e., within families, fathers are considered to be kings and mothers to be queens until women reach the age of fifty, then they also become kings (Mahmood).

Marriage appears to be less important than childbirth as a point of transition in the transference of responsibility for food-provisioning from older to younger women. Often, women seemed to reach an awareness of the importance of feeding upon the birth of the first child. For example, Monir, who had spent much of her youth in Britain, away from her family, took little interest in cooking either before or during the early stages of her marriage (relatively little childhood observation of their mothers' cooking was remembered by adult women more generally). Her mother-in-law, who lived with the couple, retained the responsibility for meal-provisioning, while Monir worked for a travel agency. However, once she had given birth for the first time she gave up her job and took over the feeding duties.

Monir – (I) just took care of the baby and did whatever a housewife is
supposed to. And it just came naturally really. …

The first birth appears to be held as a key transformatory stage in the
life span of Iranian women, and is seemingly essential for the development of mature, stable, female gender identities. It is therefore
highly significant and appropriate that they should simultaneously
take up responsibilities for looking after and, in particular, for feeding their children (and husbands), so demonstrating their attainment
of complete womanhood.

If gender roles and food responsibilities differ according to age and
life stage, female identities also appear to be variably constructed and
played out across the different regions of Iran. Azerbyjani women are
particularly renowned for their culinary prowess, as was mentioned
in Chapter 4. They are said to devote more time and attention to the
preparation of food (thereby demonstrating their excellence as wives
and mothers) than, for example, women from Teheran (who are also
more likely to work outside the home). In interviews, women from
different areas contested their relative merits in terms of the value of
these skills and the appropriateness of spending more or less time on
cooking activities. For example, some regarded the Azeris as 'too
fussy' in their meticulous food-preparation practices, other admired
and envied their devotion to such labours.

Recognition was also made of the changing nature of women's
roles and identities over time, as these are worked out in relation to
domestic food-preparation. Traditionally, in Iran, the gathering,
preparing and cooking of foods has occupied a large proportion of
women's time.

Monir – (They found) the best to their budget … that takes time, takes a
few hours a day to do that and … food is seasonal over there. You may
not be able to find a particular ingredient … unless it's in season, so
they've got to think about getting that ingredient and freezing it … This
filled their hours and their days. …

Although cooking has remained an essential task in the enactment of
Iranian female identity, as the involvement of women in paid work
outside the home has become more widespread, the amount of time
available to spend on housework has declined.

Monir – it's a bit different with me personally because, first of all, I'm
from a newer generation. The generation now … their thinking towards
this particular subject has changed a lot from say … my mother's generation and we don't really think that it's important though we still have it
at the back of our minds that this is important in the role of the family …
The emphasis is not so much on food now … the emphasis is more like

work and thinking about the future and saving up and all that, rathe
being so worried about the food.

In this study, only a small number of women I spoke to were at that
time engaged in waged employment. Although some appeared to
experience little difficulty in finding employment, in particular those in
academic posts, others were obliged to accept jobs for which they were
overqualified; for example, a former social worker is now engaged as a
factory seamstress, and an accountant is currently training as a hairdresser. Most women negotiated with their partners over the sharing of
household tasks, although one person complained that her husband
did nothing around the house, despite being unemployed himself.

Previous studies have demonstrated that their engagement in paid
labour frequently results in an increased workload for women, in that
they are expected to perform effectively in both domestic and public
spheres (for example, Counihan, 1988; DeVault, 1991: 99). In this
study, most interviewees had retained the overall responsibility for
management of the home, despite their husbands' involvement in
housework. Some voiced concern at the lack of time they had to give
to their domestic responsibilities; many reported that they had
responded by becoming increasingly efficient. A number had adopted
laboursaving strategies, although there was considerable resistance to
these in some quarters, particularly to the use of convenience foods,
which were commonly considered to be of inferior and suspect quality. Some women had also enlisted the help of their children.

> Asli – You know, when I'm working, everything is easier for me ... I must
> organise everything in time. Usually when I come back from work , I just
> make tea for the children but sometimes I (prepare in advance). Saturday or
> Sunday I make one *khoresh* (casserole) ... and then I organise for every
> night ... Every Thursday when I come home, after tea, I clean all the house
> ... sometimes (it takes) until 9 o' clock ... My daughter is 12 – she's started
> ironing ... (My son) he's very helpful ... sometimes he makes the food. ...

For women working outside the home, managing mealtimes requires
particular skill in balancing the demands and needs of all family
members. Ensuring the timing of meals to suit the needs of hungry
offspring is a major priority and one postgraduate student described
how her concern for the family and her feeding responsibilities could
not be compartmentalised, but permeated her consciousness even
whilst engaged in other kinds of work.

> Hamideh – ... When I am (at work I) just think the children are coming
> (home) and they're hungry and that's the main thing.

Even among those working outside the home and conscious of the
limitations upon their roles as housekeepers, women drew clear dis-

tinctions between themselves and English women with regard to the ways in which gender is performed through their food provisioning tasks. Many Iranians considered English women to be somewhat deficient in this respect, in terms of being less committed to their families and lacking adequate culinary skills, as evidenced by their need to resort to convenience foods.

> Leila – English women … they are not bothered about food or family. Not all but lots of them, they don't care about (the) family or food … Honestly, I'm just looking round, I don't know, but I feel if I cook … even (an) omelette (then) you can enjoy having a meal with (the) family, but English families don't. Always they use … ready food, like fish and chips, burgers … they don't bother to cook.

> Fatimeh – Do you know in Iran, the people have 3 (meals): breakfast, lunch and dinner … they … care (more) about the children than here and they like the children to have good food … Sometimes I look here (while) shopping and (see) children (eating) hamburgers and walking. I don't like this. I like, when we are eating something, to sit down together. We usually, especially on Sundays and Saturdays we have a big breakfast all together and we have lunch every day together.

Laziness and selfishness were regarded as 'unfeminine' traits and were criticised by a number of participants. However, others considered English women to be less shackled to the kitchen and family and therefore more able to pursue their own interests and to attain greater self-development. This was perceived to be a freedom which they either wished to, or else felt that they had been able to attain through living outside Iran. The idea of being able to achieve balance was highly valued by these women, that is, an ability to pursue a full and varied life in which no one aspect of their careers as women dominated.

Migration and Gender

Young people brought up in Britain are clearly influenced in their perceptions of appropriate gender behaviour not only by the models enacted by their parents but also by their exposure to British normative values, especially as gleaned from school and via the media. Girls are subject to certain restrictions upon their leisure activities and movements according to culturally specific gendered norms. However, in interviews with children and teenagers, food preparation did not appear to be clearly designated as an age-appropriate female activity or responsibility. Iranian women in Britain did not push their daughters to learn to cook, neither did they discourage boys, and in a number of cases boys showed an interest in cooking, and took lessons at school (whether or not their fathers participated in household tasks).

Overall, the views expressed by young people regarding appropriate gender roles were variable and contradictory. Sometimes the strongest role segregation was advocated by those children whose fathers took little or no part in the housework, for example two (eight to ten year old) girls who considered that cooking should only be performed by women, and that men lacked the skills required. In another case a girl remarked that her uncle's regular involvement in cooking was odd, asking her mother whether he was unhappy. In this case her own parents suscribed in theory to an equitable division of household labour, but in practice her father worked long hours and rarely engaged in domestic food preparation. Hence, it is difficult to determine whether her perceptions were influenced by the family's practical arrangements or derived from British valuations of inappropriate male and female roles.

Often, media coverage played an important part in the way young people perceived gender roles to be differently played out in Britain and Iran. Many assumed that political and structural differences resulted in Iranian women in Britain experiencing more freedom and flexibility than in Iran.

> Parvaneh – I think that Iranian people here have adopted some of the differences. They see how English people act and … Iranian men here do more housework. I think that there it's more the women who are in the house … I think it's a lot more sexist there, especially now after the revolution … from what I've seen and T.V.

Orientalism and Representations of Gender

Muslim women in Iran, as elsewhere, have been a focus of media, popular and academic attention over the last two centuries (Hoodfar, 1993). The discourse emerging from this gaze has been characterised by ethnocentric and orientalist biases regarding their inferior and subjugated status (for example, Colliver Rice, 1923: 274–80), interpreted according to western notions of 'equality' which are seen to be incompatible with longstanding Persian views of 'complementarity' (Fischer, 1979: 189). As previously mentioned, these images of Muslim women have also served to construct the oriental male (in opposition to his western counterpart) as uncivilised and ignorant, his masculinity relying on the mistreatment of women (Hoodfar, 1993). Critical Muslim feminists such as Hoodfar point out that such discourses have also commonly been perpetuated by western feminist academics. Especially in the case of Iran, with its specific forms of Islam, the failure of neo-orientalist analyses to examine other shared historical and cultural influences, as well as the role of religion, has also been problematic (De Groot, 1996: 40).

This is not to deny that gender inequalities exist in Iran, nor that they are interwoven with Islamic precepts, just as western Christian gender inequalities are bolstered by the Church (Harbottle, 1993). In fact, Islam has been a major factor in the construction of gender ideology in Iran since the seventh century, reflected and reinforced by the state through social and political channels. From an early age, children are socialised into an awareness of the significance of biological differences between the sexes as denoting key consequent social attributes (Ghvamshahidi, 1995). The legal canon, the *Shari'ah*, based on (usually male elite) interpretations of the *Qur'an* and *Hadith*, formulates the specific rights and responsibilities of husbands and wives, with the husband, as in the Christian tradition, being perceived to be the stronger and more rational partner, and head of the household; the woman's rightful place is in the home and her attitude is expected to be one of loyalty and quiet obedience (Ghvamshahidi, 1995).

In academic as well as popular discourses, there is a tendency to portray Islam as a 'lesser religion' in relation to Christianity (Hoodfar, 1993) and to overlook its positive achievements or to record the damaging effects of secular modern westernising trends upon Iranian society. For example, the reforms, including 'the Suffrage Act' and 'the Family Protection Law', introduced by the late Shah, although internationally lauded as progressive and desirable, were criticised internally as superficial. In the case of compulsory deveiling, this was inappropriate, offensive and directly damaging to some women, particularly from the lower classes, further restricting their access to the public domain, rather than leading to greater emancipation (Zonis, 1991: 108; Hoodfar, 1993). According to some observers, these reforms simply transformed existing relations of dominance, creating a modern, western version of patriarchy, in which women still remained subordinate (Ghvamshahidi, 1995). Following the 1979 revolution, there was international outrage as the Islamic regime introduced a strict dress code for women, revoked many of the half-hearted modernist reforms and excluded women from some fields of education. Nevertheless, women activists successfully lobbied for a new family protection law which afforded greater protection to women than its predecessor. More recently, a law entitling women to wages for housework has been approved by the Iranian parliament (Hoodfar, 1993). Although largely symbolic, they are probably no more so than the Shah's attempts to appease his western allies, yet in this case the measures have gone unnoticed. Instead, the international media has continued to decry the excesses of the Islamic regime and to portray images of veiled and downtrodden Muslim women. Western feminist scholars have also often disregarded the considerable successes of Iranian women activists.

> The mostly man-made images of oriental Muslim women continue to be a mechanism by which western dominant cultures re-create and perpetuate beliefs about their superiority. Moreover, the negative images of Muslim women are continuously presented as a reminder to European and North American women of their relative good fortune and an implied warning to curb their 'excessive' demands for equality with men. Yet all too often western feminists uncritically participate in the dominant androcentric approaches to other cultures and fail to see how such participation is ultimately in the service of patriarchy. (Hoodfar, 1993)

Among Iranians in Britain, the persistence of stereotyped views of Muslims and the tone of the international media's coverage of Iranian affairs since the Islamic revolution appear to have contributed to a sense of alienation from British society for many adults, as was discussed in Chapter 7. Some young people who had accepted such views found that upon visiting Iran their expectations regarding female subjugation were all-too-often contradicted and challenged by the experiences they actually encountered. Interestingly, in the following passage Shanaz, a highly educated student with little interest in cooking herself, is amazed not only by one woman's lack of involvement in domestic work, but also by the ability and willingness of her husband to take responsibility for those tasks. Despite the fact that her own father regularly cooks Shanaz finds the extent of the role reversal difficult to believe.

> Shanaz – When I was in Iran, Nila … did not do anything at all, she didn't even know how to cook and this was in the middle of Iran, the middle of nowhere. Honestly (her husband) cooked everything and she basically lazed around … The dinner he cooked in the evening was absolutely wonderful, you know, you'd think – 'really did he make all this?' … I just thought, you know, it's going to be totally male chauvinist … when I saw that I just thought it was fantastic.
>
> I was expecting … the headscarf … to have an effect on the way women were treated … but in the house I didn't actually notice it … it's just outside really, inside it wasn't a problem, it was just like being here.

Her response also underlines the point made earlier in this chapter, that is, when women cook it is a taken for granted occurrence; in contrast men performing the role skillfully and on a regular basis are seen to be somewhat exceptionally gifted.

Domestic Food-work, Power and Influence

With the evolution of feminism and the later development of cross-disciplinary gender studies, issues of cross-culturally variable gender roles and apparent asymmetrical power relations have been of central concern to anthropologists. Early analyses asserting universalist notions of male dominance and female subordination, influential among feminists in many disciplines (Ortner, 1974; Rosaldo, 1974) were gradually replaced with an awareness of gender relations as historically and culturally contingent processes, and greater sensitivity to the complex and multifaceted nature of power relations has emerged (Harbottle, 1994). Today, there remains considerable debate over the relative and different powers wielded by men and women, the conditions under which they flourish or change and their impact on the quality of social life (Counihan, 1988). Many observers have continued to maintain that sexual asymmetry exists everywhere but 'not without perpetual challenge or almost infinite variation in contents and form' (Rosaldo, 1980).

One of the key points for contention has been that of the relative separation of domestic and public spheres of activity, together with the assumption that women have lacked real power because they have had little visibility or authority in the public domain (Rosaldo, 1974). The public/private split has continued to provide a focus of debate, and a view of power as a reciprocal and dynamic force has emerged.

> Men and women, as they interact, continually negotiate the rules that define and circumscribe the specific relationship ... power is therefore not limited to its formal aspects but must be viewed in terms of a dynamic and reciprocal process. If men hold formal power, it is important to understand how women influence them to obtain their own objectives. (Rassam, 1984: 25)

Rassam concluded that in Middle-Eastern societies women were not necessarily restricted or subordinated as a result of the strictly enforced segregation practices in operation there. Others have suggested that professional Middle-Eastern women are often more independent, confident and assertive than their European counterparts, precisely because of the greater separation of male and female worlds (Fischer, 1979: 189–90). With regard to Iranian women, commentators have also noted the extent of their apparent power and status within the domestic sphere (Hoodfar, 1993) and interviews with Iranians in Britain seemed to echo this view.

> Hamideh – I mean, I think women are very powerful, I mean it's not maybe direct but it's indirect power ... you know some men ... it's because you care that they do it ... but you have to mention it to them ...

I think what I want to say (is), you have to tell them, you have to, because I think men are not very mature ... maybe they don't know very much, about, you know, love and children, and if you tell them what to do ... they care but they don't know how ... And I've heard a lot from other people that ... actually the power is in women and even you don't see from outside but it's there ... Even (if) the man looks powerful ... they're really like children. Whatever the wife ... wants is going to be.

As described earlier in this chapter, domestic food-work provides a primary means by which these Iranian women perform and reconstruct their gender identities. Counihan has, in relation to her study of Italian women (1988), argued that control of food is important because it satisfies our most basic and compelling biological needs, the fear of hunger imparting deep significance to food-provisioning. It therefore serves as a powerful channel for communication and as a means to establish connections, create obligations and exert influence.

> The predominant role of women in feeding is a cultural universal, a major component of identity, and an important source of female connection to and influence over others. Hence, although there are other components of female identity and other sources of their authority, the power of women is to a large extent the power of food. (Counihan, 1988)

She further argues that women's power over food-provisioning is not one that is coercive; at a macrolevel, for example, women generally attain little control over food availability or cost, but within households they are able to exert influential power. Mauss described how the giving of vast quantities of food on special occasions resulted in the creation of debts which the recipients were then obliged to repay (1950). Counihan further considers how gifting is carried out, on an everyday basis, by housewives engaged in the mundane tasks of food-provisioning, and she analyses how women's power is achieved, not (usually) by force and denial but through obligations created by these continual acts of giving. Hence, through the work of feeding their husbands and children, women ensure that they are needed and that they command love, respect, monetary returns and good behaviour from their families in reciprocal transactions, as well as promoting harmonious relations.

> Safieh – My husband doesn't care but I feel when I cook something which is his favourite he's happy. He shows me he's feeling better..and he eats better.

Counihan asserts that the power women obtain through food-work is largely exercised over family members and rarely extends beyond to members of the wider society. However, in the case of these Iranians, *ta'arof*, the code of ritual courtesy, includes rules determining the appropriate level of hospitality to be shown to guests, depending on the formality of the relationship (Pliskin, 1987: 53). Like the Greeks studied by Cowan (1991: 182) Iranians are expected to demonstrate generosity to guests; failure to do so indicates a lack of respect and casts a slur on the character and standing of the host family, hence, as the principal domestic food providers, Iranian women hold a vital role in maintaining the reputations of their husbands and families.

NB

> Safieh – I think that Iranian women spend a lot of time in the kitchen for cooking ... because we should have a good dinner for holiday(s) and if we invite guests to the house, we should prepare a good dinner for them. And if we don't do this it's a fault ... I think it's important for us because (we like) good food. ...
>
> Goli – The thing is food is (very) important for Iranian people ... if some-one goes to a house they expect (lavish hospitality) ... particularly old people. ...
>   I think they might ... cut down on (other) expenses to afford a good meal – they say it's *abru* – prestige.

In the British settler Iranian community women continue to follow the rules of *ta'arof*, although these are variably attenuated according to length of stay. Acquaintances are generally served tea, bowls of fruit, sweets, nuts and other tidbits. Close friends often seem to take on the role of fictive kin (Harbottle, 1995: 15) and, according to financial means and social standing, are included in more substantial food exchanges which serve to symbolise and constitute social rela-tionships (see also Theophano and Curtis, 1991: 169, and Werbner, 1990a: 259). For example, within one network of friends those who could afford to do so regularly hosted lunch or dinner parties, whilst others either held more modest gatherings or reciprocated in other ways. One woman (whose husband was a Ph.D. student) could not afford, and did not have the space, to entertain many guests but she was renowned for her baking skills and regularly provided cakes and desserts for parties.

In exchanges of food, the sheer quantity of food and the prestige inherent to particular raw foodstuffs are clearly important. However, among the Iranians I interviewed, quality was stressed as an even more important consideration, not only in catering for special occa-sions but also in everyday family food-provisioning. Even those on student grants or with low incomes stressed the importance of buying the best foodstuffs they could afford (in contrast with the predominant concerns expressed by the British women who participated in Charles and Kerr's study, for convenience and low cost, 1988: 70). If necessary, these women said that they would rather compromise on the quantity rather than on the quality of purchases.

Asli – Always it's important to me … I try to buy the best quality, like the oil, vegetables or everything. Might be I make less but I make sure it's best quality.

Even more important than the quality and freshness of raw ingredients was the sensory evaluation of the cooked dish. Iranian high cuisine is sophisticated, elaborate, colourful and rich and everyday meals also incorporate a complex and subtle blend of herbs, spices, fruits and nuts. The effort and skill invested by women is of paramount importance in determining the value attributed to the final dish and the reputation of the cook. Hence, the status held by the cakemaker previously mentioned derived not so much from the value of the ingredients she used but from her input of time, effort and skill. Her cakes conformed to the aesthetic standards valued by this group, i.e., they were considered light, well-risen, delicately flavoured and beautifully decorated.

As a further example, among Iranians rice-cooking is an art and women rate one another on their relative merits in accomplishing this skill. Perfectly cooked rice should have distinct, long, straight, fluffy grains. In this country basmati rice is usually used by Iranian women, as the finest quality and most aromatic variety available (in Iran other superior strains are preferred). The preparation process is painstaking, from the initial careful sifting to remove stones, pre-soaking (usually in the morning or the day before it is required), par-boiling and finally steaming to ensure the perfection of the final product. The addition of butter and an underlayer of potato or bread ensures the formation of a crisp layer or *tadik* which clearly differentiates Iranian rice dishes from those of other national cuisines, as do garnishes of saffron, *zeresht* and pistachios.

Through the cooking of rice and other foods in prescribed and ritualistic ways they are imbued with additional meanings, properties and values by which not only the physical, but the emotional, cultural and spiritual needs of the family (and others within the social network) are satisfied. In Chapter 6, I considered the importance of the cultural transformation of the raw ingredients wrought by the process of cooking. However, to understand the status women derive from their food-work it is important to examine more closely the meanings of the performances in which they engage.

Sered (1988) has described how the spirituality of Middle Eastern Jewish women is enacted through interpersonal relationships. For them, the 'sacred' is not compartmentalised but is deeply embedded within the 'profane' world of everyday activities. The maintenance of relationships through nurturing and caring responsibilities, such as food preparation, provides a key medium of expression and constitutes a major mode of religious experience. Similarly, for Shi'ite Ira-

nians living in Britain, although adherence to the formal aspects of
the Muslim faith is variable, participants in this study continued to
acknowledge its underlying and residual force in their lives. In contrast to secular British women for whom food-work carries no such
spiritual meaning (and carries little status), for these women, even
the most mundane tasks, such as the everyday feeding of the family,
are thereby infused with significance and importance.

From this perspective, these women's involvement in domestic
food preparation tasks may be considered as akin to the spiritual and
emotional investment involved in Christian communion rites. In the
latter case, through engaging in prayer and particular rituals, the
priest consecrates the elements and, through eating and drinking,
communicants receive spiritual fortification. Catholic theology sets
out a belief in transubstantiation, in which the substance of the bread
and wine are thought to actually become the flesh and blood of
Christ; Anglicans and Baptists argue for a more symbolic representation. However, Lutherans adhere to the notion of consubstantiation; in this case the elements are not materially transformed but are
nevertheless held to embody the flesh and blood of Christ, which are
said to be received 'with and under' the bread and wine (Richardson
and Bowden, 1983: 120–21). The notion of consubstantiation provides a useful analytical device for considering the rituals in which
Iranian housewives engage. Through their everyday and festive
cooking they also embody, concretise and dramatise central elements of culture and faith. In the process, cooked food is infused
with value and the women (or men) who prepare it, like the priests
or ministers who preside over the Eucharist, attain status and command loyalty, through the generosity of spirit and love embodied in
the processed (cooked) food.

Although the involvement of women in paid work outside the
home has increased, limiting the time available for food preparation
(and the influential power which can be exerted by this means), this
does not yet appear, as in the case of the Italian women studied by
Counihan (1988), to have resulted in an erosion of the value attributed to domestic food-work. Furthermore, although as migrants
many Iranian women are aware of subtle transformations in their
gender roles, compared to the structural restrictions operating in
Iran, they generally continue to ascribe great value to the 'art' of
cooking and to draw a distinction between themselves and English
women by so doing.

The previous chapter illustrated how Iranian men in Britain,
obliged to seek work in the fast-food trade, have as a consequence
experienced a subtle undermining of their status as men. By contrast,

this section has demonstrated how their female partners have retained their power within the domestic sphere as a result of engaging in work valued for its well'th connotations. In fact for them migration has arguably resulted in an increased valuation of that work, reflected by their enhanced status within the family. These relative shifts in gender status, together with the greater structural freedom which women experience in the diaspora, and intersecting with dominant British gender ideologies appear to be resulting in a partial and ongoing transformation of gender roles and identities.

These data also challenge stereotypical western ideas that Muslim women are subject to more overt oppression by their male partners than are their European counterparts. In fact such notions may themselves more accurately represent the projections of late twentieth century hegemonic western masculinities, under threat from the demands of western feminists. The stigmatisation and marginalisation of the Muslim other may then serve to deflect the critical gaze and to bolster vulnerable and fragile western male identities. Orientalist representations actually overlook a substantial degree of plasticity and tolerance with regard to the gender roles of Muslim men and women. To some degree these appear to arise out of a privileging and taking-for-granted of the essential importance of biological differences within dominant Iranian ideologies. Thus, although the domestic sphere, and in particular food-work, has been, and remains, primarily a source of female identity, power and status, nevertheless men are not perceived to be less masculine if they engage in these tasks.

11. CHILDHOOD, ACCULTURATION AND FOOD

The previous chapters have illustrated how the process of migration may result in the transfiguration of adult ethnic and gender identities. For the present youth generation, the hybidised cultural spaces of the diaspora may potentially offer even greater opportunities for gender malleability and fertile cultural fusions. Nevertheless, in this study, parents experienced considerable ambivalence regarding the acculturation of their children, fearing that their greater interaction with the majority population and with other subcultures, particularly mediated by their attendance at school, might lead to identity confusion among young people, or worse still to a gradual loss of their Iranian identities. Parents were more fearful with regard to girls than boys, perceiving the disjunction between British and Iranian normative gender behaviour to be more pronounced. Interviews with mothers, as we have seen, illustrated how their concerns over good childfeeding practices related not only to their attainment of sound nutritional status but also to their incorporation within Iranian culture and community. This chapter examines more closely the interrelated processes of food acculturation and identity-formation; subsequent sections then explore the identity concerns and perceptions of young people themselves, as particularly reflected by their food consumption practices.

Food Acculturation

As Fischler has pointed out (1988), not only does the ingestion of food ensure that the eater assimilates its culturally ascribed properties, but, at the same time, the absorption of that food serves to integrate the eater within a particular cuisine and culture. The process of socialisation is vital in this respect, both in terms of the formation of individual identity and the transmission of cultural values from one generation to the next. Research into the eating behaviour of young children suggests that their attitudes towards food begins to develop at a very early stage (Lupton, 1996: 37). Primary identities such as those of gender and ethnicity also begin to evolve in early childhood and studies in Britain and the U.S.A. suggest that children as young as two or three years of age have begun to internalise and reproduce ideas of ethnic variation, and may demonstrate ambivalence and/or hostility to their own or other ethnic identities (Benson, 1981: 141). There is a close interplay between the processes of food acculturation and the development of ethnic identity. Both involve the intertwining of psychological as well as social dimensions, through which individuals not only experience a sense of belonging to a group but are in turn shaped by it (Roosens, 1989: 15). Young children learn not only to distinguish between those substances which are edible and those which are not but also to recognise what counts as food within their particular cultural milieux, to define themselves accordingly and to differentiate themselves from others who eat differently. In each case the emotional charge of these early roots may contribute to their later potency (Epstein, 1978: xiv).

Fischler has noted the importance of both the symbolic and the corporeal aspects of incorporation (1988) and there has been considerable debate over the importance of physiological determinants of dietary behaviour relative to the significance of social and cultural influences. For example, an innate preference for sweet foods has been demonstrated by newborns, and infants have been shown to be able to self-select a nutritionally adequate diet (Davis, 1939). Nevertheless, children's food behaviour is generally accepted to be predominantly moulded by sociocultural, rather than biological factors (Rozin, 1989: 205).

The socialisation process starts in infancy, within the sphere of the family unit, but continues throughout the lifecycle, according to changing circumstances and influences. Although the term carries implications of passive acceptance and mimicry, in reality the individual plays an active role, demonstrating variable degrees of choice, deviance or innovation in relation to the impact of different agencies (Beardsworth and Keil, 1997: 54).

The primary feeding relationship is that established by the mother-child bond during the breast or bottle-feeding phase. From the outset, food is associated not simply with sustenance but also with sensual pleasure, intimacy and nurture (as mentioned in Chapter 3). Hence, from birth, food and feeding hold considerable emotive power which continues to underly subsequent eating behaviour.

Food socialisation begins in earnest at the stage of weaning, a process which is variably defined across cultures (Harbottle, 1996) ranging from a rapid transition from breast-feeding to family foods (*sevrage*) through to a more gradual and prolonged introduction of solids, in various stages, according to the degree of physiological maturity ascribed to the toddler within that cultural system. Cross-culturally, weaning is considered to be a time of particular physiological vulnerability for the toddler, and complex taboos and dietary regulations apply at this time (pregnant women are also subject to numerous and variable dietary constraints in order to protect the health of the unborn child).

Initially a single foodstuff, or very limited range, is introduced; as the child becomes familiarised with these tastes and textures an increasingly wide variety of foodstuffs will be made available. Young children tend to place a variety of objects in their mouths and begin experientially to learn to distinguish edible from inedible items, i.e., what is safe or unsafe to eat. At the same time they learn to discern what counts as appropriate food within their sociocultural context as they observe the responses and behaviours of parents, other relatives and peers.

Developmental psychologists have observed a range of strategies employed by parents to attempt to exert control over their childrens' eating patterns, for example, instrumental eating by which a child is promised a reward if s/he eats certain, usually 'nutritionally sound' but unpopular foods, (Boakes et al., 1987: 120). Interestingly, although parents are influential in the development of the child's personality and habits generally, Rozin suggests there is little evidence of their impact over food preferences, once the effects of culture are removed (1989: 205–9).

Generally, as children grow older they become less dependent on parental food choices and more able to take responsibility for their own diets; simultaneously peer group pressures become increasingly significant. It is not unusual for more generalised resistance to parental power to be manifested through general or specific food refusals (Brannen et al,, 1994: 151; Lupton, 1996: 56). In some cases distinct childhood food cultures may develop (James, 1979). During adolescence, conforming to group norms may incorporate the acceptance of contemporary ideals regarding body size and shape, as, for example, demonstrated over the last decade with a sharply increasing incidence of anorexia nervosa, especially among teenage girls (Lask and Bryant-Waugh, 1993). Finally, leaving home is often a time for significant dietary changes (Bull, 1985).

Dependency to Autonomy? Iranian Settlers and Food Acculturation

As we have seen, in traditional Iranian cosmology, and within other humoural systems (see, for example, Tan and Wheeler, 1983) the importance of maintaining hot-cold (*sarde-garme*) equilibrium is much greater for the young child, who is considered to be less tolerant to changing conditions than are adults. In this study several mothers considered that toddlers, and more particularly infants, were especially prone to 'coldness' and they attempted to maintain their good health by dissolving a small amount of *nabat* in their childrens' feeding bottles.

Although few of these women adhered closely to *sarde-garme* beliefs at other times, in their infant-feeding practices they appeared to draw more heavily upon traditional recipes and lay wisdom. Notably, these women generally displayed considerable confidence in their ability to adequately feed their children. This contrasted with previous research findings among predominantly second generation, and less affluent South Asians who appeared confused by contradictory advice given by health professionals and family members (Harbottle and Duggan, 1992).

Although a detailed nutrition survey of this group has not been conducted, the observations I made and discussions held with mothers indicated that these women's lay wisdom and infant-feeding practices generally seems to accord with current nutritional recommendations (with the exception of the addition of sugar to milk feeds). Colostrum was considered to be very good for infants, and was not discarded as is common practice among some other Muslim groups where it is deemed to be dirty and polluting. Solids were rarely introduced before the age of three months, although fruit juice would commonly be given earlier. At the three to four month stage some form of gravy, soup or broth was often introduced, the texture gradually becoming more solid as the child became accustomed to chewing.

> Soraye – I started with (meat) juice. I always put it in the pressure cooker (with) onion (and) cook(ed) it really well. Everyday I gave her 1–2 tsp of juice. Then gradually, I added green lentils, rice, parsley … I put them in (the) food processor (and gradually increased the quantity).
>
> My mother says lentils and rice and parsnip and coriander, and when they are older, spinach – these are good … After one year (I) started feeding her (an) adult diet.

James (1979) has argued that childhood is a liminal phase, during which the development of specific childhood food cultures may be used by young people to mark their position and to maintain a degree of integrity outside the adult order. Although her argument is very convincing in relation to British society, its relevance to non-western societies, in which individuation is not so highly valued as a normative process, is more questionable. Certainly, from these interviews, it would appear that in Iran, once the weaning process is completed, children eat the same foods as adults. Similarly, there was no evidence among Iranians who had recently arrived in Britain of special foods being consumed, or of established childhood food cultures.

Nevertheless, in the case of families who had resided in Britain for a longer period, there is some indication of what appears to be the development of new social categories and of the establishment of distinct differences between childrens' and adults' food habits, (although there were no apparent gender differences at this stage). This seems to be moderated primarily through the impact of the childrens' peer group. Hence, young people who had lived here for a considerable length of time had adopted certain habits, such as the regular consumption of sweets and chocolates, a preference for easy to chew, modified meat or fish products, for example, fish fingers and chicken nuggets, and foods such as chips, beans, spaghetti hoops, and sweetened breakfast cereals, specifically targeted at this market niche. However, rather than identifying designated 'childrens' foods', parents are often asked for 'English' food and in this way the difference between parental and youth cultures is affirmed.

Asli – (My) children don't like Persian food, (they ask for) English food 'especially (at) the weekend, they ask me to 'make the English food'.

Mehri – When I ask them ... 'what will we have for lunch today' and I (suggest) rice and meat 'oh not again ... I like fish and chips ... because I'm English now' ... I just laugh, I don't listen to them ... They like Italian food, pizza (and) macaroni. ...

In this study, parents often talked about Iranian identity as if it was something vulnerable, which could be easily lost and they were explicit in their recognition of early childhood as an important time to begin the process of instilling Iranian values, for example, through appropriate diet and language training (Harbottle, 1995: 20). Nevertheless, adults acknowledged that if they wished their offspring to prosper and to achieve upward social mobility, they would need to conform with the majority culture and with their own peer group. Mothers apparently negotiated and compromised over the menu-planning with their children (and in some cases there was a considerable degree of contestation). Commonly, they agreed to prepare English and other ethnic meals on some days, provided that Iranian dishes were consumed at other times (the elements comprising British cuisine will be considered in the following chapter).

However, not all children were keen to eat British food, as illustrated by one account in which a child, separated from his parents and looked after by his siblings, expressed his longing for his mother's presence by rejecting the meals prepared by his brother and sister.

> Monir – I remember one time ... my mother ... left our younger brother with us ... He was about 8 or 9 and he went to school, so we were kind of responsible for his food, and we kept feeding him with burgers and, you know, these quick ready-made foods ... And he was quite used to having ... fresh foods – proper foods – made for him. So one evening this poor child he was fed up and he started crying his heart out, saying 'I want my mum back. I've not had proper food for so long' ... this became a joke when my mum got back. And my older brother was so taken aback ... that he started trying to make rice. ...

This account demonstates the affective potency of food as a source of security and familiarity, and reiterates the importance of the symbolic aspects of incorporation. Despite the presence of other family members, this child missed the love and nurture provided by his mother; the daily offering of foreign food did not therefore satisfy his appetite, although it may have met his energy requirements.

Iranian Youth, Food and Identities

According to Caplan, there has been very little direct focus by anthropologists on the food consumption practices of immigrants and ethnic minorities in Britain (1997: 13). Rather, such work has proceeded mainly from a nutritional perspective (within which biological notions of race remain prominent) and has tended to focus on diet-related disorders, such as diabetes amongst specific (usually black) groups (for example, Cruikshank and Beevers, 1989). The anthropological focus on the food habits of minority youth cultures is even more sparse, although there have been a number of studies of other aspects of cultural production within diverse populations (for example, Yates, 1990; Amit-Talai and Wulff,1995; Back, 1996).

Much of the contemporary literature on cultural identities has been generated within the politics of race discourse (Back, 1996: 4) and this present chapter draws insights from that field (for example, Hall, 1990), as well as from feminist theorists who have drawn attention to the diversity and partiality of identities (for example, Haraway, 1990; Strathern, 1991; Moore, 1994). From these perspectives, identity is perceived to be subject to a process of formation and flux, according to changes in the life cycle, political institutions, social relations and the degree of authority a person attains (Hall, 1990: 222; Rutherford, 1990: 24). The importance of class, gender, sexuality and religious differences within and transecting ethnic boundaries have been recognised and Derrida's term *différance*, which infers a suspension between 'to differ' and 'to defer', has been usefully employed by some authors in an attempt to signify the transformative nature of diaspora identities (for example, Fischer and Abedi, 1990: 253–56; Hall, 1990: 229–35).

In relation to the cultural dynamics of everyday life, Yates's study of British Muslim girls makes the point that whereas indigenous white youths may develop only a minimal consciousness of their ethnicity, Muslim girls have to work much harder to develop a sense of ethnic identity, because he argues, they exist in a 'frontier culture of contested meaning' (Yates, 1990: 87). If this is the case, then the importance of food as a means of establishing and modifying cultural identity may be of much greater significance for minority groups than for the ethnic majority. Yates's work is also important in relation to these data in that he considers the complexity of the intersections between religion, sexuality, family relationships and future expectations with an awareness of ethnicity, and he draws attention to the ways in which the girls engage in a series of cross-illuminations from one arena to another. Nevertheless, his understanding of cultural systems as 'tectonic plates' and the dualistic experience he imputes to the girls' lives, in their creation of identities which could withstand pressures from 'two cultural milieux with the minimum stress' (1990: 81) implies rigidity and stasis in both dominant and minority cultures.

Back, in his recent ethnography of urban youth cultures (1996) attempts to move away from this kind of absolutist analysis. He seeks to locate cultural production within the context of both global and local influences and engages with the plurality of minority ethnic identities, at the same time interrogating dominant codings of what it is to be British (Back, 1996: 4). This 'new ethnicities' approach more closely resonates with the findings from this study, in which it is apparent that both English and Iranian cuisines and cultures have been profoundly inflected by transnational influences, including those of invasion, migration, trade and tourism. Like the Londoners studied by Back, young Iranians living in multicultural cities in Britain, are not situated between two mutually exclusive and primordial cultural systems, being tugged in two opposite directions. Rather, the ethnicities from which they select elements are already plural and multivocal. However, Back's consideration of the selective inhabiting and vacating of social identities, according to changing circumstances and agendas conjures up images of tangible and

permanent structures, as well as inferring the relative separation of
those identities (Back, 1996: 124). These data suggest that the performance of ethnic identities by young people is more flexible, pol-
ysemic and inflected by other roles.

Considering the development of a black youth culture among
Surinamese migrants in Amsterdam, Sansone makes the point that,
comparatively speaking, cultural identity may be considered to be
more flexible among younger members of a group than among older
people (Sansone, 1995: 126). Certainly, in this study, interviews with
parents indicated that they considered their childrens' identities to
be more vulnerable than their own.

> Naser – That's the problem, you know, identity is always a problem, not
> for me – for my children – she is British or she is Iranian. Everybody has
> got this problem. we used to come and study, go back home ... we are
> Iranian, that's it finished. but now it's different with the kid ... when she
> grows up, she doesn't know she is British or Iranian, that's the difficulty.

In this account, and in other interviews, parents tended to draw upon
essentialist understandings of ethnicity and often seemed to perceive
their children as caught 'between two cultures' (Watson, 1977). Werbner argues that this process of self-essentialising is valuable as a
means of imaginatively maintaining moral and aesthetic communities (1996: 312); it has also played a major role in mobilising groups
to political action (Hall, 1990: 223). It is therefore important that any
analysis of cultural production, including food consumption, incorporates a recognition of the sustained importance of the notion of
bounded and pure identities in people's lives, as well as theoretical
consideration of inherent difference, diversity and contestation.

However, although the Iranian participants in this study often
drew upon imaginary notions of stable, continuous and bounded
cultural systems, the cultural milieux in which the older generation
were socialised, in Iran, has not been static but is itself a hybrid
blend, encompassing a number of foreign influences. The process of
migration has also led to transformations in ethnic and other identities and in some interviews this was also acknowledged. Indeed,
Naser, who implied his own identity to be stable and unproblematic
in the passage above, later went on to observe – 'I'm almost like (the)
English I've been here so long'.

Nevertheless, in addition to the multivocality of their culture of
origin, the present youth generation appear to have been more
exposed (primarily through their participation in the education system) to a diverse range of local sub-cultures, and therefore have
potentially greater opportunities for reinterpretation and 'play' with
cultural forms. The liminality of their position, in relation to the lim-

ited structural constraints placed upon them, is also important in this respect and may allow young people considerable scope to eclectically tailor their cultural, and other, identities as will be explored in the following chapter.

Childhood is a key period in the development of food habits and identity-formation, and the primal roots formed then carry great potency in later life. This chapter has illustrated how these processes are interrelated, and has shown how, for British Iranian children, as for other minority groups, the diaspora community is one in which modifications to both culture and cuisine are ongoing and complex. The apparent emergence of new social categories and of distinct childhood food cultures is perhaps the most marked of these changes. For the present youth generation, their early exposure to a multivocal parent culture, and to a diverse range of local subcultures, facilitates manifold opportunities for a reinterpretation and 'play' with cultural forms and gender expression as we will now consider.

12. PICK 'N MIX CULTURES
YOUTH, FOOD AND IDENTITIES

This chapter focuses on the accounts of four teenagers (two male and two female – selected from a wider group of participants) and highlights the considerable flexibility and complexity in their understandings of ethnicity and other intersecting identities, including gender. It explores how these are reflected in their food consumption practices and further considers how the paradoxical tendencies towards both novelty and tradition, which are evident within food cultures, may be of varying significance over the lifecourse. Whereas earlier chapters have emphasised the tendency of women, while performing food-provisioning tasks, to attempt to maintain a sense of culinary coherence and continuity, and men to engage in the defensive strategies of dissimulation and pretence, this chapter illustrates how young people act as the primary cultural and culinary innovators within their families, and considers the longterm impact upon British Iranian cuisine.

Hassan

Hassan was fourteen years old when interviewed. He was born in Teheran, but brought up in a provincial town. He came to Britain in 1992 with his parents and his younger brother and will shortly return, when his father completes his period of study. Hassan is now settled in the local secondary school, although it took some time to adjust. In particular he found it difficult to relate to girls in the class. In Iran, a gradual awareness of the differences between the sexes had been sharply reinforced by a physical separation of male and female schoolchildren, from the age of six. Unaccustomed to their presence, Hassan had felt awkward when he had been put in a mixed class in Britain.

> Hassan – I think it shouldn't be like that because you don't get an idea of
> what people are really like … (you) don't really get to know them that
> well, so you don't know what to say.

He also hinted at some problems with children who had mocked
him for his accent, his religious beliefs and his diet; indeed, there
have been cases reported of ethnic minority children rejecting or
'forgetting' to take their own food to school because of the attitudes
of their peers (Mares et al. 1985: 92). However, in his mother's presence Hassan was keen to play down the importance of these events
and to emphasise the value of supportive relationships in counter-
balancing racist or unpleasant behaviour.

> Hassan – there's a few (unpleasant people) now but I've got loads of
> friends, so it's OK. I'm not bothered what people say.

At the time of the interview (which followed a T.V. documentary on
the economic plight of Iran, considered to be very biased by a number of interviewees) Hassan was more concerned that Iranians were
misrepresented through the media and preoccupied with the impact
this had on his friends and acquaintances. The conversation flowed
from consideration of the oddities of different cuisines to the ways in
which food habits and whole cultures could be misrepresented by
those who lacked understanding.

> Hassan – Iranian food is misrepresented on T.V. … Asians and people
> from other countries are usually misrepresented as second or third class.
> On T.V. they only show the poor, not rich – if they do that they should
> show the poor in America as well.

Hassan has a quiet, serious and polite demeanour. It comes as no surprise when he states that religion became personally significant to
him at the age of eight, not, he says, through the impact of religious
studies but 'when you see other children, you know, fasting, it strikes
you' (196: 85–87). Asked to describe early memories of food he draws
upon nostalgic recollections of celebrations of the Muslim holy day.

> Hassan – usually we'd go on Friday to my dad's brothers … and have
> kebabs or whole lamb on the spit, roasted … It was the day off school.

Hassan started fasting occasionally in Iran but, influenced by other
Muslim pupils at school, he began to take it more seriously and
recently completed the whole of Ramadan (one month). Influenced
by his mother's concern to maintain her family's Shi'ite identity
(described in Chapter 6) as well as his own preferences, Hassan eats
predominantly Iranian foods, made with halal meat and/or recipes
modified by his mother. If Hassan's friends come for a meal, his
mother usually finds out whether they'd like to try Iranian food; if

not she serves adapted versions of preferred dishes. On rare occasions, the family may eat out, in which case a local Iraqi restaurant is preferred, or a pizza restaurant or takeaway. Hassan used to eat at McDonald's but gave up, perhaps surprisingly, not because of the use of non-halal meat, but because of the B.S.E. scare – 'they say they're importing the beef from another country but you can't always believe them'.

From his contact with schoolfriends, Hassan views the English diet to be generally limited with lots of ready prepared meals. Asked about the most important aspects of the Iranian diet, he commented on the significance of rice; bread may be more commonly eaten (in some parts) but rice has more prestige and is essential with special foods like *ghormeh-sabzi*. He was especially struck by the contrast between the painstaking and complex process of rice preparation in Iran with the way it is cooked in Britain.

> Hassan – it's really funny because it's in a plastic bag, that's just how I saw people cooking it, and I was surprised at first. ...

A dominant motif within Hassan's account is the moral stance he holds against the unnecessary killing (i.e., other than out of the necessity to eat) or infliction of suffering upon animals. This concern may intersect with his religious beliefs to some extent and/or may be influenced by his peer group. Hassan's account illustrates something of his gender, religious and moral, as well as ethnic, affiliations. Although he considers himself Iranian, he is aware of the impact of his stay in Britain, and of the difficulties he will have in readjusting when he returns to Iran.

Ali

Ali was sixteen and attending a GCSE college when interviewed. He came to Britain in 1991, at the age of eleven. In contrast to Hassan's parents who are keen to maintain their sons' Shi'ite beliefs to ensure their smooth transition back into Iranian life upon their forthcoming return, Ali's parents intend to stay in Britain and are overtly more liberal, with religion appearing to hold a residual, rather than a prominent place in their lives. Ali himself has a very different personality from Hassan. He is lively, boisterous and he seems to more closely resemble a rebellious British teenager than Iranian norms for a young man (at his age classed as an adult). This is expressed through his conformity to peer group norms, in terms of his musical taste, his involvement in sport and social activities, and with regard to the conflict in his relationship with his parents. It would be easy to assume from a superficial encounter, that Ali is more adjusted to life in England and to assume that a sense of Iranian identity would hold less valence for him.

However, his food behaviour gives some indication of his individual sense of identity. He claims to 'eat anything' and is not fussy, liking takeaways, popular Italian dishes and, having been familiarised by a school visit to a Chinese restaurant, he also requests his mother to make Chinese dishes; still he prefers and more usually eats Iranian food. Despite lacking conceptual knowledge regarding the Muslim faith and the differences between Shi'ism and Sunni factions (and in spite of active discouragement from his mother who was concerned that he should not be impaired in his GCSE preparation) nevertheless Ali considers it important to fast during Ramadan. Interestingly, he has a number of Pakistani friends who also fast and give him encouragement, yet he sees Ramadan as an occasion to mark his identity as specifically Iranian.

> Ali – It's like thanking God for all the food and ... a way of thanking Him and appreciating all the goodness he's given us. And I do fast ... I did it recently – the whole of Ramadan ... having said that, I have to do that because I'm almost 16 and I have to follow (the) religious (laws).
>
> It's one of our traditions in Iran. I'd like to (stay) Iranian, be Iranian, follow Iranian traditions as much as I can, no matter where I am. And this is one of the easiest ones. Some of the Iranian people I know, they hardly know about Iranian culture because they've been born here or they've been brought up here from childhood, so ... I'm not criticising or anything but they've missed out. I mean it's something extra knowing about Iranian culture.

Although Ali doesn't have much more factual knowledge regarding the beliefs he holds than those whom he feels have lost out, he has a sense of having retained an Iranian ethnic identity in a form extraneous to his everyday involvement in British culture. Rather than seeing himself as occupying an ambiguous and uncomfortable position, he sees the advantages of his situation. However, for most of the time ethnicity and talk of food are not on his agenda, 'I mean especially at my age, it's the last thing we talk about'.

Parvaneh

Parvaneh was also sixteen and studying for her GCSEs at the time of her interview. Her family came to Britain in 1985 and her dietary preferences suggest that over time she has been increasingly influenced by the majority food culture.

Parvaneh – I have to say I prefer English foods because we have so much Iranian food, you just get a bit sick of it, so I prefer English food. And chicken is my favourite – but we do eat Persian food.

Her family still have Iranian main meals on three or four days a week. However, on other days they eat Chinese, Indian, Italian or English food. Parvaneh was the only interviewee who had had close contact with an English person who cooked 'traditional' English, rather than international or fast food. Parvaneh's mother had obtained a number of recipes from her; the family particularly enjoyed roast dinners, shepherd's pie, leek soup and yorkshire pudding!

For Parvaneh, McDonald's was a favourite place to eat out because other friends congregated there. Rather than selecting Middle-Eastern restaurants as in the case of the previous two families, if Parvaneh's parents took them out, it was more likely to be to an English restaurant. Parvaneh draws a distinction between these eating places and the pubs frequented by English friends' families.

Parvaneh – I love going out for meals. We sometimes go out as a family, to a restaurant … it's usually (to an) English … restaurant … But when I go out with my friends and their famil(ies) it's (to) a pub usually.

Parvaneh considers herself a Muslim but is not religious and she doesn't know anything about Muslim beliefs.

Parvaneh – To tell you the truth I know more about Christianity … I go to a Christian school (because it's a good school). I hear about that more … but I am a Muslim.

She also thinks of herself as Iranian but, having been back recently for a visit, acknowledges that she would not fit into the way of life in Iran.

Parvaneh – I wouldn't like to move back, not with the government being as it is. If it was as it was before the revolution, I'd love to go and see what it was like … I don't feel at home anywhere really. When I'm here I'm treated like a foreigner. When I'm there I'm treated like a foreigner because I've been here since I was 5 so I just make the best of it really. Most of the people at my school just treat me like one of them.

In this conversation she seems to express views which fit with the notion of ambiguous culture, of being a foreigner both here and in Iran, yet when she talks of her friends it is clear that her ethnic identity is not always something which is problematic. Rather, in close relationships other identities, such as age and gender, become more important. She later goes on to consider the advantages of being bicultural and of being able to incorporate selected aspects from each. Indeed she is able to command the respect of others for her knowledge and cosmopolitanism.

Parvaneh – From the age of 6 I knew two languages and I think that's quite an advantage. People look at you as if you're really clever ... I like the (variety of foods too) I think it would be quite boring ... if it was all English or all Iranian. My mum makes different food(s).

Shanaz

When interviewed, Shanaz was seventeen and had lived in Britain since the age of three. She had recently started at University and was living in a shared house, with four other students (all English). Shanaz had never cooked before, to the surprise of housemates, who expected her to be skilled in the kitchen (in fact, only one of the students is able to cook well and they generally eat separately).

Shanaz – (W)e don't really see each other that much ... but I've noticed that we all seem to live on pasta – it's easy to make ... occasionally we'll have rice ... but it always seems to be tinned food and soup or spaghetti or something, but nobody actually bothers making a meal or anything like that ... Only once, we've had a Sunday lunch.

The thing is I've not really learned how to cook properly ... because during my 'A' levels, I was so busy on my work that food was just there on the table ... That's what everyone was surprised (about). 'Oh, you come from a foreign background but you don't know how to cook'!

Shanaz's diet is now strongly influenced by the need for quick and easy meals and she tends to make use of convenience products. Like many other young women (Brannen et al., 1994: 153) she does not like red meat and although she eats chicken, she tends not to buy it because of the mess and inconvenience of preparation. She also skips meals and has a rather erratic pattern of intake, practices which generally appear to be more common among females than males (Bull, 1985; Brannen et al., 1994: 104–5). In particular, Shanaz usually misses breakfast, due to lack of time, and either takes fruit with her, or buys chocolate mid-morning. She may make a sandwich for lunch, or buy something from the university canteen, usually pizza, pasta or fish and chips. Her diet now is markedly different to the one she followed at home, provided by her mother. Then, mealtimes were regular and on most days Iranian dishes were consumed at the main meal of the day. At the weekends, takeaways such as pizza or fish and chips would usually be eaten (for example, following the Saturday Farsi class).

During the interview it became clear that food is not a major concern in Shanaz's life at present, as she responds to the new challenges of her degree course and social life. As she reflected upon her former eating habits, it also appeared that her education has been the main priority over recent years. The support provided by her parents is symbolically represented by the fact that, despite the importance of the shared family meal, during her 'A' levels Shanaz sometimes ate alone in her room, and was waited on by her mother so that she could continue to revise without distraction.

Just as sojourners returning from trips to Iran bring with them foodstuffs as a tangible reminder of the care and support of the family at home (as mentioned earlier), so Shanaz's mother has similarly attempted to maintain family and cultural ties with her daughter. On one visit she brought some *ghormeh-sabzi* (Shanaz's favourite dish) hoping to ensure her daughter would eat properly. Instead, the food was put in the freezer and forgotten about as Shanaz immersed herself in her studies!

In discussing university life and her adjustment to a new lifestyle, she articulated a strong concern over the pressure to drink alcohol. The importance of alcohol commensality in public social events in many cultures has been noted (see for example, Gefou-Madianou, 1992: 6). Although Shanaz considers herself a Muslim she does not practise the faith. Yet, not having been socialised into an alcohol-consuming culture, neither has she developed a taste for this innately unpalatable substance (Rozin et al., 1986: 98; Lalonde, 1992). At university she was initially perturbed at the extent to which social events involved alcohol and found it difficult to cope with the pressure from others to drink, and the resultant feeling of exclusion if she resisted.

> Shanaz – I don't really tend to drink at all. I don't really like it. At first I found it a real problem ... because everybody expects you to (drink) and they couldn't really understand why I didn't. And I had to say, it's not the religious side ... they (think) because you're a Muslim you can't drink ... but (it's not that) ... I'm not really that fond of alcohol ... I'm happy with a soft drink but, yeah it is a big thing ... at uni you have to drink otherwise you're not considered one of them ... I think it's very big but I try not to let it get on top of me and people accept that I don't want to drink. But, sometimes, when you meet new people (they ask) why not? ... We tend to be in the pub all the time in the evening.
>
> At first they thought I didn't want to mix with them but I think they've grown to accept it.

The subject of taste aversions was more fully elaborated in Chapter 3, but in this case what is particularly interesting is that Shanaz's aversion to alcohol arises not from her religious convictions but from cultural norms in which drinking is not modelled as desirable behaviour, so that the habit is not readily acquired through socialisation. Her friends apparently find it more difficult to understand and respect this justification for not drinking than that of religious motivation.

For most of the time, it would appear that Shanaz's role as a student has taken priority over other possible identities. Significantly, because of her academic commitments, she has missed out on the recent annual *No Ruz* celebrations (perhaps the most culturally significant calendrical event to Iranians). However, she has recently met another Iranian student and together they have considered aspects of their cultural backgrounds and current identities.

> Shanaz – I have thought about it quite a lot. It's something that's always on my mind, you know – how should I be? English or Persian? I've not come to a conclusion ... I still think of myself as Iranian but possibly I think I've an English attitude. Sometimes my dad says to me 'that's an English way of thinking' ... I think sometimes my dad thinks you can't do that because you're a girl, you have to be a boy to do that. I just think how can that be. Boys and girls are supposed to be equal. ...

Although she is not a practising Muslim, in her account there appears to be a degree of fusion between culture and religion and a powerful intersection between gender and ethnicity. As an Iranian (Muslim) teenager, a number of restrictions have been placed upon her movements and social life. However, these have, to some extent, been counter-balanced by the family's desire for social mobility and belief in the importance of educational achievement, resulting in their encouragement of her pursuit of a professional career. Their consequent acceptance of her leaving home has resulted in a transition, with Shanaz now being given greater autonomy and responsibility for her own actions.

Pick 'n Mix Cultures

In the past studies of cultural identity have often tended to imply fixity and stasis and to overlook a focus on other intersecting identities. In this respect the reconceptualisation of identities as affinities, allowing for attachments which are 'contradictory, partial and stategic' has been valuable (Haraway, 1990: 197). Affinities are less rigid, more fluid and allow scope for change, thus resonating more with the eclectic 'pick 'n mix' approach which Iranian migrant youth are able to take in relation to their identities and food preferences.

These findings illustrate how ethnic identities may be modified according to exposure to different cultural systems, to the extent that new social identities may evolve. In particular, the emergence of the life-stage 'teenager', with its overtones of emotional lability, appears to be novel for Iranian, as for other non-western migrant families in Britain (Leichty 1995: 179 and 191; Brannen et al., 1994: 41). In this study, Hassan illustrates the Iranian model of a non-individuated development to adulthood, in which adolescence is a period of physical maturation but is not seen as a process of emotional separation from one's parents. At fourteen years of age, he is responsible, courteous, and conforms readily with his parents' wishes and requests (Pliskin, 1987: 55), as well as with their eating patterns. Ali, on the other hand, appears to be engaged in a more ruptured progression to adult status, and is experiencing the turmoil more in tune with British adolescent norms, which is perceived by his parents to be problematic. He is much more independent in terms of when, as well as what, he eats and he is less willing to compromise with his mother over meal planning.

The teenagers interviewed here clearly hold a number of different social roles simultaneously, in addition to their polyvocal ethnic identities, and these may be variably reflected through their food consumption practices. They may be regularly or occasionally performed (or may be imaginary) and there is no necessary consistency or logic to these, although some identities intersect and interplay with one another. For example, the case studies show how gendered experiences of adolescence vary; Shanaz and Parvaneh are marked by their female identities, so that they are subject to certain restrictions upon their movements and a greater burden of parental responsibility, regardless of their age.

These accounts also illustrate how gender and ethnic identities are further inflected by age, lifestage and geographical location. In this study educational achievement was highly valued, to the extent that the occupation of scholar significantly modified other (in particular gender) roles and at certain moments appeared to subsume other categories (for example, during preparation for major exams, or the first year at university). In Shanaz's case, moving away from home becomes an important transition point, at which she is able to achieve independence from her parents, as dramatically reflected by her change in eating habits.

Culinary Boundaries and Diffusions: Reflections on British Food Cultures

In addition to the observations made by Shanaz regarding the importance of alcohol in university social events, the interviews highlighted other key aspects of British food culture. Firstly, and most prominently, few of the young people had clear notions of what comprised 'English' cuisine.

Shanaz – (I)t's funny, when I was in Germany (on a school exchange trip) I was asked that question and I really couldn't think. All I could think of was fish and chips, I didn't really know what typical English food (was) … The lady I stayed with in Germany, she asked me that and I was … stuck for words … The girls in my house, they tend to eat … it's not typically English or anything. (One) is fond of Indian food and she makes hot stuff.

Ali – Things like (roast) beef, fish and chips and generally that sort of thing. I don't really know to tell you the truth because … at other peoples' houses, when I go for tea, they're often having a takeaway or something.

Fish and chips were commonly mentioned, by parents and young people alike, as the epitome of British food culture and a favourite meal. Ironically, there has been a sustained and considerable immigrant involvement in their production (as was discussed in Chapter 7). Nevertheless, the consumption of fish and chips has been described as:

perhaps *the* culinary sign of Britishness, it has been nationalised as much as socialised, with the result that it now tends to suspend rather than expose fundamental sociocultural distinctions. (Adair, 1986: 49)

Apart from fish and chips, interviewees were generally familiar with, and sometimes ate roast and/or Christmas dinners (but not usually puddings). The Sunday roast and, more particularly, the Christmas dinner carry great symbolic force (Douglas, 1982) and the inclusion of these elements of English cuisine by Iranian settlers is therefore significant. However, generally, participants seemed to perceive British food culture to be relatively simple and unelaborated, and as one teenager remarked 'I think English people like all nationalities' food because they haven't got any' (Shirene). In this way British and Iranian cuisines were often contrasted and the boundaries between them were marked.

The uncertainty with which interviewees refer to British cuisine seems to resonate with its failure to impact significantly at an international level (particularly in the light of the widespread influence of the empire and the global dominance of the English language). This may be related to the British emphasis on saving time and money (Mennell, 1985: 260) and their perceptions of food as a necessity rather than a pleasure. Hence, although British expatriates may have clung tenaciously to familiar dishes, rarely have they persuaded others to adopt them, and even the exports of prestige foods, such as kippers and stilton cheese are relatively small (Driver, 1983: 92). This may also explain why other cuisines have held such sway in Britain. By contrast, in France, with its more highly elaborated food culture and indulgent attitude towards eating, although Indo-Chinese and Chinese cuisines have made some impact, national traditions have apparently been retained to a much greater extent than in Britain (Mennell, 1985: 330).

The accounts of these young people highlighted the profound recent impact of international cuisines upon British food culture (Driver, 1983: 73: Warde, 1994) to the extent that one interviewee considered chilli con carne to be 'English' food (Ayesha). This dish is reportedly a bestseller in one supermarket chain, along with other international dishes such as lasagne and chicken tikka masala (James, 1997: 71). They also reflected recent transformations such as the increasing consumption of convenience and takeaway foods (Johnston, 1977: 127; Mennell, 1985: 330).

As well as asserting boundaries between English and Iranian food, several people showed concern that their friends had confused Iranian with Indian cuisine and expected it to be hot and spicy. 'Most English people think of it as being a curry ... it looks like a curry but it tastes nothing like it (Parvaneh).

> Hassan – I'm sure people used to think ... you know, it's really hot but when they've tried it out it's not that hot.

> Ali – They go like, 'do you eat a lot of curry' ... 'no I eat different foods' ... and that's it, end of conversation.

The fact that these young people drew my attention to their friends' confusion over culinary boundaries also appeared to overlay a common anxiety that they themselves might be assumed to be of Indian or Pakistani origin; this anxiety was also expressed by a number of adults previously interviewed (Harbottle, 1995: 21).

> Parvaneh – They tend to think anything outside of Europe as being either 'Paki' or something like that and because Pakistan and India and Iran ... are around the same area, they just think of us as one type of people.

Interestingly, despite the popularity of Indian food amongst the ethnic majority, it was not highly favoured by most Iranians interviewed. Even those people with Indian or Pakistani friends and who had eaten in their homes were not keen on hot curries; in some cases more marked aversions were demonstrated.

> Shanaz – My Pakistani friend from school, she tends to have hot food every day. Once I had dinner at their house and I remember thinking – how am I going to eat this. I thought it's just going to go straight through me. (My brother) ate curry and it made him sick.

Capsaicin, the active pungent agent in chillis, is an irritant which causes increased gastric secretion and gut motility, however these physiological responses and the initial innate dislike of the substance are commonly overcome through social conditioning (Rozin et al., 1986: 98). However, in Shanaz's apprehension regarding the effect of this curry on her digestive system and her brother's actual episode of sickness, there may be evidence, not only of an absence of conditioning to the substance, but perhaps also of a stronger fear of the effects of its incorporation at a symbolic level (Fischler, 1988).

Chillis are often consumed raw or pickled by many Iranians, with subtly flavoured stews or kebabs. However, the combined heat of the chilli with very pungent curry spices creates a distinctive 'flavour principle' (markedly different from the flavour principles characteristic of Iranian cuisine which were described in Chapter 4). This apparently serves as a powerful marker of Indian food and is associated with Pakistani and Bangladeshi groups, subject to strong negative stereotypes in Britain. Hence, this food aversion may reflect a reticence of Iranians to assimilate aspects of these cultures, which might further devalue their own status within British society. Additionally, the rejection of Pakistani identity may have historical roots in the self-perceptions of Persians as superior to Indians and Pakistanis and in the opposition between Shi'ite and Sunni sects of Islam.

In sharp contrast to the unfavourable response to Indian food, Italian cuisine was generally very popular among young people and adults alike in this study and often seemed to provide a useful bridge between British and Iranian food cultures – pizza, lasagne and spaghetti, in particular, being served up to schoolfriends from any ethnic background.

> Shanaz – There tends to be a lot of Italian restaurants ... and everyone likes the food ... I think it caters to everybody's (taste) ... I don't know anyone who doesn't like Italian food.

The widespread acceptance of Italian food also accords with the attempts by Iranians in the fast-food trade, described in Chapter 7, to pass as Italians in order to protect and disguise their own identities. Perhaps by eating Italian food there is also a hope of enhancing their own ethnic identities and of achieving greater acceptance within wider society. Certainly these data support the argument made in Chapter 3 that taste serves as a metaphor by which the organoleptic properties of food connote the relative symbolic values ascribed to different cuisines and cultures according to different contexts.

Novelty and Tradition: Cultural Hybridity and Food Consumption

The foregoing accounts have demonstrated something of the complexity and fluidity of diasporic Iranian youth cultures and how this may be reflected through food and eating. Youth is a transitional

and liminal period during which there may be considerable freedom
to 'play' with identity-formation, but this may not necessarily be sustained in later life. At present, there are few adult second generation
British Iranians and it is therefore difficult to determine whether the
kinds of hybrid culture celebrated by these youths will endure with
maturity or whether these youngsters will 'revert' back to reliance
upon familial and ethnic networks.

Certainly, evidence from Werbner's study of Pakistani settlers suggests that their integration into British society and culture is very partial in adulthood, with little joining of voluntary associations which are
not ethnic. According to her, young married Pakistani adults tend to
return to the fold and to embrace South Asian popular culture, clothing, cuisine and language, rather than engaging in other voluntary
activities shared by the ethnic majority (personal communication).
Nevertheless, some Iranians argue that they are more accommodating
and less resistant to outside cultural influences than are South Asians.

> Mahmood – We have dropped our fashion ... and we have imitated (oth-
> ers) ... We have been influenced by so many cultures that (we've got a)
> sort of mingled – amalgamated culture ... we are very adaptable, very
> hospitable, very respectful to foreigners. ...

Academics (for example, Fischer and Abedi, 1990: 253; Hoffman,
1990) have also remarked that Iranian culture has been subject to
rapid and remarkable transformations in recent years, and if the culinary culture of young Iranians in Britain is as malleable as these
commentators suggest then the modifications observed in this study
may well be of considerable and lasting significance.

However, too much change at too rapid a rate, as Warde has
pointed out (1997: 57) may lead to personal and social disruption.
Fischler has also described the 'gastro-anomy' resultant from a
breakdown in the long-standing rules governing food intake, which
he considers to be a feature of contemporary modern society (1988).
This threat may lead to defensive strategies such as an increasing
appeal to 'tradition' and the invocation of an imaginary, continuous
and coherent community (Warde, 1997: 58). However, a common
problem in postmodern studies of consumption and cultural hybridity is that in their preoccupation with the ephemeral and contingent
aspects of identity-formation, they have lost sight of the ideological
significance of 'pure' and bounded categories; what is needed is a
processual theory which effectively encompasses both and which
explores the moral battleground between cultural purists and innovators (Werbner, 1997: 3–4, 12).

In this respect Bakhtin (1981) offers insights which may develop
our understanding of the paradoxical coexistence of the trends

towards 'tradition' on the one hand, and novelty on the other, evident within the food consumption practices of these Iranian migrants, as well as within the majority food culture (Warde, 1997: 57). In his studies of linguistic hybridisation, Bakhtin draws a key distinction between a superficial, conscious, and intentional hybridity and an unconscious, deep 'organic' hybridity which he argues is a feature of the historical evolution of language (1981: 358). Despite an illusion of boundedness, cuisines are also gradually (organically) transformed over time through a series of 'unreflective borrowings, mimetic appropriations, exchanges and inventions' (Werbner, 1997: 5–6).

Bakhtin's distinction offers a useful means by which to consider the food cultures of Iranian youths in Britain. At a conscious, aesthetic level, these young people clearly engage in a certain amount of play with signs, especially the visual signifiers associated with style, fashion and taste – for example, when they eat out with friends or select school meals. Consumption studies have predominantly tended to focus on this intentional manipulation of signs, yet they are probably of relatively superficial and short-term importance in the formation of individual identity (Warde, 1997: 203). Other more deeply rooted and unconscious aspects of self-identity, such as emotional security and a sense of belonging are also implicated in food consumption practices.

As well as individual identity-formation, the incorporation of food also serves to construct collective identities. Warde describes the process by which the development of a group identity is 'less a matter of personal zeal, more the becoming immersed in a Bourdieuvian habitus – deep-rooted subconscious, informal, given, persistent' (1997: 183). Bourdieu's (1984) notion of habitus does not, however, adequately develop the potential for transformation. Bakhtin's analysis of organic hybridity more effectively explains the process of long-term and gradual modifications which do not disrupt the existing sense of order and continuity within a cuisine.

Throughout its history, Iranian food culture has been continually shaped by its contact with a number of invading forces including the Chinese and the Turks (Zubaida, 1994a: 33–48), as well as by trade contacts with neighbouring states, and, increasingly, by global influences, but it has retained a sense of coherence and continuity. Such changes are often integrated unconsciously, for example, in the case of Iranians who have settled in Britain, the use of raw ingredients produced under different growing conditions, minor variations in traditional recipes according to the availability of ingredients, and reductions in fat intake in response to contemporary health concerns, are the kinds of food modification which are largely imperceptible.

Similarly, new themes may also be almost indiscernably encompassed and claimed as Iranian by subjecting them to Iranian cooking
techniques, or by slight modifications in the ingredients – for example, the recipes for spaghetti (with *tadik*, – a crusty layer) and pizza
(made with halal meat and green beans – as described in Chapter 6).

Werbner asserts that organic hybridity creates the foundations
upon which intentional or conscious hybridity builds, to challenge,
revitalise or disrupt (1997: 6). In this study, not surprisingly, young
people were more active as cultural innovators within the family
unit, experimenting with new foods (and fashions in music and clothing) at school and requesting these at home. It was also apparent that
mothers, through their daily food-provisioning tasks, were primarily
responsible for building stable cultural and culinary foundations and
for maintaining a sense of coherence and continuity within their families' food patterns. Thus it appears that the domestic food tasks of
Iranian women in Britain are of considerable importance in maintaining a sense of relative cultural stability and in providing the ontological security needed to permit their children to engage in playful
and eclectic food consumption practices. In the process new and
diverse culinary elements are gradually woven into existing culinary
repetoires, so revitalising and transforming British Iranian cuisine.

This chapter gives voice to Iranian teenagers in Britain and
demonstrates that the potential multivocality, contradictions and fluidity of plural identities are perhaps most profoundly experienced by
the present youth generation. Through their flexible 'pick 'n mix'
approach to food consumption they are able to variably perform a
range of ethnic and other identities. The long-term significance of
such 'play' is not yet clear for this group but these findings do suggest
that many of the elements currently introduced on an experimental
basis, will be modified and incorporated within British Iranian cuisine as it continues to evolve. The chapter also further enhances our
understanding of the significance of domestic foodwork in maintaining a sense of culinary and cultural coherence, and in explaining
why women derive considerable respect and status through their
performance of these everyday tasks.

13. CONCLUSION

Migration, Food and Identity

Identities, as this text has demonstrated, may be understood by those who claim them, to arise from essential attributes (especially those based upon bodily features such as sex characteristics). However, such bodily features are themselves assigned significance only in a social context. Social identities are thus created, and are moulded, contested and modified in the flux of social interaction, encompassing the performance of a wide range of everyday activities and roles, including those of food-provisioning and consumption practices. Although culturally determined rules frame the enactment of a specific role, nevertheless each actor draws upon his/her own experience and interpretive capacity during a particular performance, allowing considerable scope for transformation.

As we have also seen, identities are not simply a matter of internal definition but are forged in an ongoing dialectic interplay between internal processes and external referents. Thus, for example, although the majority of Iranian men in this study were highly qualified and they may have considered themselves to be intelligent, diligent, forward-looking and ideally suited to many professional occupations, in Britain they commonly found themselves to be defined otherwise by British employers and fellow employees. Potent stereotypical labels, for example 'ignorant', 'backward', 'religious bigots', conflicted with internal processes of identification and in order to preserve positive identities, these men sought ways to minimise the impact of externally imposed definitions, for example by adopting strategies of dissimulation and pretence, as was observed among workers in the fast-food trade.

As the substantive chapters of this book have also demonstrated, the relative significance of internal and external processes of identification is not constant but varies according to the relationship of the actors with the wider society. In this study of Iranian settlers in Britain, it is clear that the potency of external processes of categorisation varies according to the structural positions of men, women and children and the extent of their contact with the majority population, resulting in differing opportunities and constraints in the performance of key social roles, in particular that of ethnic identity.

These data have further shown that, in contrast to the ethnic majority who may be largely unaware of their processes of identity-formation, for ethnic minorities such as these Iranian migrants, identity issues may become more urgent and at times may be problematic, especially if there is significant dissonance between the beliefs, values and practices of the host and settler groups, or within the internal-external dialectic. In such a context, the urge to maintain their ethnic identities may be increased. Moreover, the study has highlighted how transfigurations of ethnic and gender identities may be brought about and reflected through changes in the performance of social roles, including those associated with food-provisioning and commensality. For example, in the previous chapter we saw how Shanaz, rather than attaining female adult status through the culturally sanctioned route of marriage and childbirth (as in the case of her mother and the majority of that generation), was able to achieve independence by her adoption of the role of scholar. For Shanaz, the successful performance of this role seemed to involve, and perhaps even to require, her exclusion from activities more traditionally associated with the enactment of ideal female Iranian identities, in particular cooking. Her performance of the role of scholar/student continued to be modified and reinforced in the university environment as she adopted the actions and behaviour of her peer group, including skipping meals, snacking, and the selection of ready-to-cook or simple meals, rather than choosing to 'cook properly'.

Her social behaviour leads us to the conclusion that there is considerable flexibility and scope for the reconstruction of her multivalent identities. However, simultaneously, it is clear that Shanaz perceived limits to the extent to which she could modify her identities and this belief was also reflected in her behaviour. For example, although she participated in the social activities of her peer group of students, including outings to public houses, her involvement was delimited by her embodied resistance to the consumption of alcohol. In this way she continued to ensure that she was ascribed as 'other' within the group and she simultaneously reinforced processes of internal identification by which she considered herself to be Iranian.

Although in this study young female identities were generally not marked by the acquisition and practice of cooking skills, older married women's food preparation tasks within the domestic sphere were very important in the assertion of their gender identities and in the maintenance of individual and collective Iranian identity. As I have argued, the significance of these tasks has to be understood in relation to the key concern of Iranians to maintain the health and wellbeing of their families. I have also demonstrated that within Iranian cosmologies the spiritual, cultural, nutritional and aesthetic elements of feeding are not regarded as separate concerns but are enmeshed within a holistic view of 'well'th'. An understanding of Iranian cosmologies and a research approach which combines analysis of the symbolic with a recognition of people's understandings of the functional dimensions of food and eating is vital in illuminating why women's domestic food-work, generally considered in Britain to be of low status, is highly valued by both men and women within this emergent diaspora culture.

As I have argued, Fischler's theory of incorporation (1988), which recognises that we 'become what we eat', both through metabolic processes and through our absorption of the symbolic signifiers assigned to specific foodstuffs, is crucial to this analysis. It is primarily the cooked meal which carries symbolic valence in terms of identity-formation and, adopting a modified version of Lévi-Strauss' culinary triangle, I have theorised the significance of the cooking process in relation to the potential cultural transformations wrought. Much of the value intrinsic to the meal lies in this cooking process and in the aesthetic and emotional activities of the cook. Despite this fact and the acknowledgement of the skills required to be a professional chef (Fine, 1992), with the exception of Sered's (1988) valuable contribution, consideration of the actual tasks performed by domestic cooks has been largely overlooked by social scientists and nutritionists. Yet, it is clear from the present study that the performative aspects of women's feeding-work – the preparing, peeling and chopping, cooking, garnishing and serving – together with the investment of time, love, and consideration during each of these stages, imbue food with cumulative layers of meaning. By engaging in their cooking rituals women facilitate the reincorporation of the eater (who, by eating, assimilates the emotional investment of the cook along with the food) into Iranian culture and cuisine. Simultaneously, in the performance of their roles as cooks and nurturers, women reaffirm and reinforce their status as female members of their community.

Iranian women in Britain are faced daily with the threat of negative incorporation from food they perceive to be contaminated by a variety of toxins, which, I have further suggested, symbolise the immorality and negative values of western society. These women are able to address their dilemma by engaging in specific culinary performances by which they apparently reclaim food perceived to be denatured and so make it edible. In this context it appears that the migration process results in an enhancement of women's status, as their food-work becomes increasingly significant in the reinforcement of their families' health and cultural identities.

As I have illustrated in this ethnography, the importance of women's food-work in the home needs to be contextualised in relation to the position of those Iranian men employed in the catering trade. Whereas the domestic food-work of migrant Iranian women apparently bolsters and enhances their own gender status and their families' Iranian identities and demonstrates the importance of internal processes of identification, men, by contrast, derive little respect or status from their public food-preparation tasks. Their work more clearly highlights the potency of external aspects of the identity dialectic. For these men the work itself is not central to the performance of their gender identities, rather its primary importance lies in the economic exchange-value it commands, as reflected by commercial food sales. It is this which facilitates their performance of other relational roles, in particular, husband and father, which are important in maintaining their respect and status as men. Nevertheless, their socioeconomic advancement is circumscribed by wider structural constraints and the employment of men, who are often highly educated, in relatively unskilled work, and in a sphere largely associated with women and other migrants, diminishes their status within their own social group to some extent. Furthermore, the fact that this work involves defensive rather than proactive strategies (for example, the attempts to pass as Italians or Greeks), as they engage in a disguise, and thereby a protection of their internalised cultural identities from external labelling, may also undermine their standing, particularly in relation to that of their wives.

Whereas the data derived from interviews with women emphasised the importance of maintaining Iranian identity through the provision of familiar food (and other aspects of cultural production, such as language training), and particularly stressed the concern that their children should not lose their Iranian identity, information obtained from young people themselves provided a different perspective. This illustrated how they negotiated, came to terms with and benefited from their multivalent identities. In this case the relationship between internal and external processes of identification appeared to be more compatible and equitable, leading to opportunities for positive cultural fusions and reproductions, rather than to stagnation or retrenchment. Although there were apparently moments of high tension, fraught with ambivalence and ambiguity, during which they perceived themselves to be caught between two very diverse cultural systems (and cuisines), generally the younger generation seemed to enjoy a considerable degree of latitude to engage in playful performances of their ethnic identities, which included what, with whom, and in which setting they chose to eat. Interestingly, however, such play does not extend equally to all cuisines and Iranian youths, like their parents, appeared to be very reticent to consume Indian (encompassing Pakistani and Bangladeshi) food, and were eager to draw a distinction between themselves and other Muslim groups discriminated against by the ethnic majority.

The eclectic cultural performances of Iranian youth may be partly attributed to their liminal position, according to which young people are relatively free of the structural constraints experienced by their fathers as members of the British labour force. These youths were less inhibited in their interactions with their peer group and were able to playfully enact a range of identities or affinities (including ethnic identity), in contrast to the cultural 'passing' practised by Iranian men. These diverse types of performance may also be associated with different aspects of identity-formation, the 'play' of young people seemingly being more reflective of superficial, transient and individualistic processes, while the affective urgency underlying men's need to 'pass' perhaps represents more deep-rooted and long-term elements of social identity-construction.

Warde (1997: 203) has recently criticised the predominant focus, in contemporary consumption studies, on the more individualistic and relatively superficial aspects of identity-formation (particularly the emphasis on the visual signifiers associated with style and status) and the relative neglect of collective aspects of identity-formation. Data from this study have highlighted how the individual and the collective are commonly entangled and implicated with one other and have further demonstrated the need to embed analyses of style in a broader consideration of the way food may be implicated in other aspects of identity-formation, including emotional security and collective belonging.

The convergence and relative significance of the two dimensions – i.e., the superficial style-associated elements, and the long-term, deep-rooted and collective aspects of identity-construction – is perhaps most clearly depicted in the study by the menu-planning performances of mothers and their children. Accordingly, through repeated processes of contestation, negotiation and compromise, mothers work to ensure the continuation of a diet which they consider to be broadly

Iranian and which reinforces the collective identities of their families.
Simultaneously young people are able to experiment with a range of
new foods and culinary themes outside the home, some of which are
gradually integrated within the domestic meal-cycle. Through these
interactive performances an organic and cohesive process of culinary
modification emerges, encompassing long-term subtle changes, as well
as more pronounced short-term innovations. In these food-related
exchanges, women and children assert and at the same time transform
their individual and collective identities.

Food-work, Health and Gender Status

As I have argued, by engaging in their domestic food-work, Iranian
women in Britain carry out the important and valued work of maintaining the health and cultural integrity of the migrant family. In the
process they attain positions of respect and status within the family
and the community. Ironically, Iranian housewives not only attain
higher status than the majority of their British counterparts through
their food-related activities, but they also command greater respect
within the community and from their male partners than professional food and health workers (particularly dietitians) obtain from
their medical colleagues or from the general public.

This may be related to the fact that, in Britain, the hegemonic biomedical model of health continues to privilege a curative approach
and has been less concerned with the maintenance of good health,
encompassing wider aspects of wellbeing (which I have incorporated
in the notion of well'th in this thesis). This may be one reason why
the well'th connotations of domestic food-provisioning have not
been highly elaborated or valued. In contrast, within traditional Iranian frameworks health-care (with food preparation as an integral
component) is considered to be an everyday and vital observance.
Because it is regarded as highly important work, those (usually
women) who enact the role of health guardians also attain particular
respect and status.

A useful analogy of the contrast between British and Iranian valuations of food and feeding-work in relation to their associated cosmologies of health is provided by two cult figures within ancient
Greek mythology – Hygeia and Asclepius. Hygeia was the guardian
goddess of good health and Asclepius was the male god representing
curative medicine, whose cult eventually replaced that of Hygeia.
Together, they may be understood to symbolise an 'oscillation
between preventive and curative medicine' (Dubos, 1992: 7). The

myths of Hygeia and Asclepius also illustrate a power struggle between male and female roles in health care and food-provision. In Britain, the hegemonic role of biomedicine (historically male-dominated) and its association with 'advanced' technologies and 'powerful' drugs coincides with a devaluation of other more mundane and easily accessible forms of treatment, in particular diet therapy. Pharmacists (mainly male), dealing with industrially manufactured drugs, frequently enjoy higher status within the biomedical system than dietitians (predominantly female) and are constantly consulted by hospital doctors, frequently with regard to matters of nutritional import.

Moreover, the Hygeia/Asclepius myth underlines a further opposition – between technical competence and aesthetic value. Within biomedicine the former has been privileged and even within sociology little attention has been paid to the aesthetics of work, the focus being directed instead to technical, functional, relational and goal-directed aspects (Fine, 1992). This is also reflected in the nutrition field – dietitians have attempted to move away from the artistic associations of their work and to transform their collective image in order to demonstrate that their technical/scientific competence is equal to that of pharmacists.

Ironically, within the domestic sphere the devaluation of the creative and sensory components of everyday food preparation may account in part for the low status with which it is generally accorded in British society. Nevertheless, the nurture, comfort and enjoyment produced by an attractively presented and tasty meal may have immense consequences of health and well-being, as demonstrated in this study. Paradoxically, the creative and artistic skills of male professional chefs are highly valued in our culture, whereas the relatively unskilled nature of food-work in the takeaway industry apparently contributes to its low status. Clearly then, no simplistic associations between the gender of the worker and the status of the work can be made, rather the interrelationships between food and public/private; male/female and technical/aesthetic oppositions are much more complex and worthy of further research.

The Potential Value of Anthropological Perspectives to Nutritionists

Although a symbolic approach is central to this study, it does not fall into the trap, common to earlier and more tightly-bounded symbolic analyses, of overlooking the significance of the corporeal significance of food and eating (encompassing peoples' nutrition cosmologies and perceptions of their bodily need for food). Neither, as in the case of nutrition science, does it privilege the functional dimension at the expense of the sociocultural and political aspects of food and feeding. Rather, this ethnography has attempted a more holistic consideration of the importance of food to a specific group of migrants. In exploring the food consumption practices of Iranian settlers in Britain the study also serves as a mirror, reflecting back upon and giving insights into the cultural valuations of food and feeding by the ethnic majority and by health and nutrition professionals.

As a former nutritionist, I found the ethnographic research process led to considerable personal reflection upon the history, assumptions, research agenda and methodological approach of that discipline and resulted in the identification of a number of areas which would benefit from cross-disciplinary dialogue and exchange with anthropologists. For example, nutrition surveys are commonly undertaken to establish the prevalence of specific nutrient deficiencies or disorders. However, they are very expensive, time-consuming and often cause considerable inconvenience (and sometimes discomfort) for the participants. In this ethnographic study my observations suggested that Iranian women feed their children well (and in accordance with current nutritional guidelines). Therefore, the likelihood of a significant level of malnutrition related to problematic feeding practices was very remote in this group. The inclusion of a pilot ethnographic phase of research, during which a simple check-list of nutritional risk factors could be applied (Harbottle, 1999: 218–27) would provide an effective means of ascertaining whether there was adequate justification (both ethical and financial) to proceed to a more invasive full-scale nutrition survey.

The inclusion of an exploratory ethnographic phase would also potentially enhance the cultural sensitivity of the researcher in relation to the group being studied (Harbottle, 1996), and would thereby improve the data-collection process, and also, conceivably, the cost-effectiveness and pertinence of the research project. Furthermore, as I pointed out in relation to my own research, even in cases where nutritionists are able to identify and to establish the prevalence of particular nutrient deficiencies, their methodological tools do not facilitate an understanding of the reasons for, or meanings of, food practices within a particular social context. Inclusion of anthropological perspectives and methods would highlight the significance of, and provide the means of eliciting precisely this kind of data, which is vital to nutrition education attempts.

In fact, one of the most important aspects of the work of nutritionists is the prescription of a 'healthy diet' and the education of the public in this regard. However, nutrition education efforts generally underestimate the significance of 'culture' in food choice and eating behaviours. Instead, they tend to be based upon an individualist 'lifestyles' model which comprises a single person's habits, attitudes and values (Blaxter, 1990). This popular health education model also overlooks the impact of structural factors upon food choice and perceives a relatively unproblematic relationship between information transfer and the decision to practise healthy eating (Davison et al., 1991). This often results in victim-blaming, whereby individuals are judged to be responsible for their own poor health. However, anthropological and sociological perspectives demonstrate how food consumption fulfills broader social functions, including the delineating and legitimating of social differences. Awareness of these analyses would better enable nutritionists to understand why individuals are resistant to complying with dietary advice, and would perhaps lead to a modification of current approaches.

Ironically, although cultural factors are not widely perceived by health professionals to be of major import with regard to the food consumption practices of the ethnic majority, they are thought to be of considerable significance in relation to minority food habits. However, in this respect 'culture' is understood in a somewhat reductionist way, and often amounts to the focus on a small number of 'cultural considerations', including religious beliefs, dietary prohibitions and dress restrictions. The convergence of the victim-blaming biomedical ethos, with the nutrition focus on problems, together with this reductionist application of 'cultural factors', then tends to result in the representation of ethnic minority diets as deviant and of their cultures as problematic (Pearson, 1986: 47). Recommendations aiming towards improved outcomes are then based upon the assumed desirability of nutritional assimilation; these have rarely proved to be effective in improving health outcomes (Bhopal, 1989). However, anthropological studies of ethnic minority groups, such as Okely's *Traveller Gypsies* (1983: 81–83) have demonstrated that attempts to enforce assimilation are subject to resistance and contestation, which may be reflected by a strong degree of adherence to traditional health practices and food habits. Advice given by health professionals which promotes nutritional assimilation, while demonstrating ignorance of lay food beliefs and alternate health systems, is shown by such studies to be inappropriate and ineffective in producing the desired changes. In terms of a policy approach, this is clearly a waste of resources. Moreover, it ignores the profound importance of food and eating in the construction, maintenance and transformation of cultural (and other) identities and it therefore fails to consider the meanings and significance attached to specific foods and eating practices. By contrast, this study has illustrated how food is integral to the construction of social identities, and how processes of cultural and culinary transformation are far more complex, contextual and contested than has been recognised by nutritionists. If nutritionists are to achieve greater success in changing the nation's diet, nutritional expertise must be matched by a deeper understanding of the sociocultural significance of food and eating.

As I have stated previously, the integration of both micro and macro perspectives is essential to a holistic analysis of the significance of food consumption practices. For too long nutritionists, and indeed nutritional anthropologists, have focused solely on individual households and communities, often resulting in temporary or partial solutions to problems which are actually rooted in structural inequalities. This thesis, although primarily engaging in a micro study of Iranian Shi'ite settlers in Britain, has demonstrated how local food consumption practices are impacted by, and need to be analysed in relation to, global trends and power relations. In particular, I have illustrated how western political intrusions and pervasive cultural infusions in Iran have resulted in anxiety among Iranians (even those living in diasporic communities) regarding the dangers of west-toxification. I have proposed that this fear is reflected in attitudes to food and eating, and in the daily food preparation tasks of Iranian women in Britain.

I have also shown how the Iranian revolution has had a pronounced effect upon British perceptions of Iranians in diasporic communities and upon the ways in which they conduct their social lives, and food-related work within the public sphere. Not only do Iranians face structural disadvantage as a non-white ethnic minority group, moreover their Iranian national identity is marked in very particular ways according to the stereotypes arising from international responses to the Islamic revolution. The lack of impact of Iranian cuisine upon takeaway or restaurant food cultures appears to be attributed to their reaction to these externally imposed stereotypes, as well as to self-stigmatisation, such that Iranian entrepreneurs seem reticent to expose their food to further probable rejection. Thus it is clear that the meanings and uses of food within societies are subject to, and intersect with, wider cultural, political and economic processes.

Whereas nutritionists, and indeed nutritional anthropologists, have largely taken a politically-blind approach and they have rarely considered the global relations of dominance underlying food consumption patterns, there is, for the future, a need for further engagement with these dimensions which continue to result in gross inequities in

access between 'first' and 'third' world nations. Analyses of the interests, behaviour and effects of development agencies, multinational
corporations and other involved institutions and actors could also be
undertaken. For example, it is now common within the field of nutrition, as within biomedicine generally, for food and pharmaceutical
companies to finance research projects, fund conferences and support
prominent individuals who will serve their interests. The construction
and dissemination of knowledge is therefore shaped in very specific
ways. Nutritionists involved in their everyday activities are generally
too immersed in the scientific discourses propagating such knowledge to observe how different sets of interests may be played out
according to the status and power wielded by the protagonists
involved. However, dialogue with anthropologists and an awareness
of social constructionist perspectives might bring about a more reflexive and critical assessment of the scientific endeavour.

Nutritionists would also benefit from a more reflexive awareness
of their own social positioning and status in relation to the groups
being studied, and of the implications with regard to the data
obtained. For example, in my former capacity as a nutrition
researcher I noted that many South Asian families who were
approached by us refused to take part in that study. Through discussions with the project fieldworkers, I gradually came to realise that
some people were suspicious that our real intention was to gather
information to pass on to immigration officials. Many were also reticent to participate in research which they believed would lead to the
reinforcement of existing stereotypes (Harbottle, 1996). Whereas,
within biomedicine, the encounter between the researcher and the
study participants is generally assumed to be a politically neutral
one, anthropologists recognise that the research relationship tends to
reflect and to some extent to reproduce an existing social order. For
the future, nutritionists would do well to consider how their research
may reinforce existing inequalities, before planning and embarking
upon such programmes.

Perhaps one of the key differences between anthropological and
nutrition approaches is the willingness of anthropologists to listen to,
to engage in dialogue with, and to learn from, rather than simply
seeking to uncover facts or to disseminate information. Ultimately,
the respect of persons, of their worldviews and collective lifestyles is
perhaps the most important and powerful tool within the research
process, whether anthropological or nutritional. As this book has
clearly shown, individuals and groups within a society do not simply
maintain existing food habits because they are ignorant, primitive or
stubborn (as is often assumed by nutritionists), but because food is

integral to the socio-cultural fabric of their societies, and specific food consumption practices are charged with multiple layers of symbolic and material meaning. In the case of this particular group of Iranian Shi'ite migrants, it is apparent that although beliefs concerning the physiological properties of food comprise a significant determinant of food choice, exploration of these without an accompanying analysis of the wider cultural aspects of food and feeding would be wholly inadequate. As this text has demonstrated, within diasporic communities the symbolic valence of food appears to acquire even greater potency, offering as it does a key medium for the delineation and transformation of primary social identities such as those of gender and ethnicity.

APPENDIX
BRIEF METHODOLOGICAL DETAILS

Study Timetable

November 1993–April 1994: Exploratory field-work phase

This was initially designed to serve as an ethnographic pilot phase for a combined nutrition and anthropological study. At that early stage I had intended to focus specifically upon the weaning beliefs and also upon the actual dietary practices of British Iranians. However, during interviews a number of themes recurred, relating particularly to issues of identity, and these gradually emerged as key focal areas of study, as described below. Simultaneously, my own awareness of and interest in the symbolic aspects of food consumption increased and I decided to pursue these topics in more depth and therefore to engage solely in ethnographic data-collection.

At this stage the field was centred around South Manchester (to which I commuted) and encompassed a small group of Iranian Shi'ites (who were long-standing friends) and their social networks. Initially weekly day trips were made to establish contact in a research context, gradually, as the level of confidence in the study increased visits became longer. However, this often relied on the willingness of participants to invite me to stay and I was very conscious of the need not to outstay my welcome, so that individual visits rarely lasted more than four days. Field work comprised participant-observations within homes and at social gatherings such as parties and picnics, as well as interviews with each of the participants. As I was generally treated as a guest my participation in domestic food-work was largely restricted to setting the table or clearing away and occasionally washing-up. I was frequently present during meal preparation (and was expected to stay to eat) but was only rarely permitted to assist and then only in unskilled tasks such as washing salad ingredients or shelling nuts.

In this preliminary phase it became apparent that women, who were generally responsible for food-provisioning within the home, seemed to be regarded as guardians of the health and ethnic identities of their families. Meanwhile, a considerable proportion of Iranian men (i.e.,75 percent of male contacts in this preliminary phase) were involved in public foodwork, i.e., were employed within the fast-food industry. The two spheres of domestic and public food-work appeared to form discrete lines of enquiry, and I felt the analytic process would be more effective if the field-work was divided into distinct phases which first focused on each domain of activity separately, and then considered both types of work together in relation to the gender identities they articulated. At this stage I identified a number of research themes which were to form the basis of interviews and observations during each subsequent phase of the field work:

1. Exploration of the links between health, identity and domestic food-work.
2. Analysis of the factors motivating Iranian men to enter the takeaway food trade and of the apparent failure of Iranian cuisine to impact upon the ethnic food sector.
3. The contrast between the apparent respect obtained by Iranian women for their domestic food-preparation and the relatively low status held by their male counterparts, and the disjunction between these and Orientalist gender stereotypes.

January–June 1995: Fast-food and restaurant field work

The exploratory field work period had been based upon interviews and participant-observations in homes and at social gatherings which were also mainly centred around the home. This phase had generated a considerable amount of data regarding domestic food-work, but had not ventured into the public sphere of commercial food-preparation. I decided to pursue this subject before conducting more field work based on domestic food-provisioning. This was partly in order to better contextualise each set of data in relation to the other and also because I felt so immersed in, and familiar with, the data generated within the domestic arena that I needed to create a distance from them in order to achieve greater analytical clarity. I also felt that the division of the field work and analysis in this way would make the writing-up process more manageable and would allow insights gained from one phase of field work to be tested and modified in subsequent stages. I therefore opted to follow each data-collection period with an analytical and writing-up phase before proceeding to the next topic of investigation.

By this stage I had decided to expand the field geographically rather than simply seeking other participants from within the Greater Manchester region. This was partly for ethical reasons – those interviewed in the preliminary phase easily recognised other participants, despite the use of pseudonyms, and there was some concern at the possibility of political repercussions. Given the level of mistrust between Iranians of different ethnic, religious and political affinities, and the need to be known and trusted by the community in order to gain access (as observed by Hoffman, 1990) it also seemed unlikely that I would easily obtain a heterogenous sample within a single geographical location. Additionally, I had established contacts in Sheffield and more recent links with Iranian families within the Stoke-on-Trent area and a number of them had expressed interest in the study and wanted to be involved.

From this stage onwards interviews provided the primary source of data, with participant-observations mainly providing supplementary information, which complemented and corroborated interview accounts and sometimes generated further questions for investigation. During this phase employees of fast-food ventures were interviewed in their homes and/or places of work. I also observed interactions between employers, staff and customers and made participant observations in one establishment in which I worked as an unpaid employee on several occasions. Although useful in reinforcing and contextualising the interview data, the need to concentrate on food preparation and service tasks to some extent hindered the observation process and the exercise was not particularly profitable in terms of generating new avenues of enquiry. Moreover, these takeaways were largely staffed by Iranian men and my entrance to this predominantly male sphere of activity resulted in a change in these men's behaviour towards me, and at times resulted in some discomfort in my relationship with these participants so I did not attempt to repeat the experience.

In discussing their selection of occupation, some employees in the fast-food trade mentioned that they had considered the restaurant sector but had decided that Iranian food would not be marketable. Since I found Iranian cuisine to be highly palatable I was intrigued to discover why it has not achieved the popularity of other ethnic cuisines, for example, Thai food. I made several participant-observation visits to one Iranian restaurant in Manchester (the only one apparently flourishing in that city). At first I visited in the company of other Iranian diners, then with an English friend, and later alone. Finally I made a visit to interview the proprieters. However, I found it almost impossible to obtain data by which to compare and contrast these findings; apparently none of the other restaurants in the North and Midlands which had been mentioned to me were still in existence. At this stage I felt that a trip to Kensington (reportedly the best established Iranian community in the country and the site of a number of Iranian restaurants) was necessary. A friend advised me that he knew a well-known and respected Iranian businessman in London who would be happy to introduce me to a number of restaurant owners. Although I repeatedly postponed the visit for over two months I was unable to make contact with this businessman and (unsure of his willingness to help) I eventually decided to make the trip alone. I spent two days in Kensington, drinking coffee, eating meals and snacks and talking to street sellers, shop owners and restaurant staff. Although a number of people were friendly and willing to talk, others were distinctly hostile and I felt that the absence of a trusted patron undermined my ability to gain access. Rather than make repeat visits I further tested my findings by discussing them with Iranian contacts and academics who lived in and around London and who were familiar with recent changes in the restaurant scene there.

July-August 1995:

Analysis and writing. Return of transcripts to participants for feedback.

August-October 1995: Domestic food-work and health

More in-depth interviewing and additional observations were made during this period, particularly focusing on everyday (rather than festive) food-work within the home. Both women and men were interviewed during this phase, although observations predominantly focused on women (I saw only three men cooking everyday meals at home). Through their daily cooking performances it appeared that women enacted and reinforced their roles as women, wives and mothers and so commanded considerable respect for their work. My observations generated questions concerning the ways in which Iranian men and women understand the relative positions of the sexes and how they articulate these beliefs in practice, in particular the extent to which they consider food-preparation to be gendered work. These questions were to form the basis of the next phase of field work.

October-December 1995:

Analysis, writing and feedback.

December-April 1996: Gender relations

At this stage participants were observed as they performed their relational and occupational roles. Interviews were conducted with men and women, together and separately. This was intended to be the final phase of field work until the reported comments of a young girl made me realise the need to incorporate the views of children and teenagers.

May–July 1996:

Analysis, writing and feedback.

July–October 1996: Field work with young people

Although children had been involved in all of the social occasions in which I had participated, until this stage I had not really 'seen' them. As a result, this chapter relies predominantly upon the interview data obtained at this late stage in the data-collection.

October–December 1996:

Analysis, writing and feedback.

Research Participants

I include here only those individuals interviewed in relatively formal situations, and from whom I collected demographic details. In more informal interview situations, such as those conducted without prior acquaintance (in particular the interactions with stall owners, shop keepers, takeaway and restaurant staff in London), I felt this would be deemed an unnecessary invasion of privacy which may have jeopardised the research process. Similarly during participant-observations I did not generally record such details. I have chosen to refer here to interviewees by a numerical coding rather than to apply the pseudonyms given in the text. This is because I found that the amount of detail included in my Masters' dissertation allowed participants to identify one another easily and a number of individuals were concerned that outsiders might use the information for political purposes. For the same reason I have withheld other identifying features, such as region of origin, current geographical location, ties of friendship, business connections and the links between gatekeepers and other research participants, in order to ensure that individual profiles are sketchy and therefore difficult to identify. Although my response to their concerns may be considered to be overcautious, I feel that the interests of the research participants must remain my paramount concern. Hence, the list which follows is necessarily incomplete, nevertheless it does give an indication of the demographic characteristics and of the social range encompassed by the sample as a whole.

The list of participants is divided into four sections which connote each of the key research questions successively explored within the main phases of field work – i.e., the high level of involvement of Iranians in the fast-food trade, yet relative invisibility of that cuisine; the importance of domestic food and health work; the significance of food-work in the construction of gender identities; and the significance of childrens' food consumption practices in processes of identity-formation. A number of individuals took part in more than one phase of field work, thus some details are repeated.

Fast-food/restaurant focus

1. Male takeaway employee and part-time mature student, forty years old, single, lives alone, born in Iran, has lived in Britain for twenty years.
2. Male takeaway owner, forty-two years old, married to 16, lives with wife and one child, born in Iran, has lived in Britain for twenty years.
3. Male food wholesaler and entrepreneur, forty-five years old, married to 17, born in Iran, has lived in Britain for eight years.
4. Male takeaway owner, forty-one years old, married to 18, lives with his wife and two children, born in Iran, has lived in Britain for twenty years.
5. Male takeaway owner, forty years old, single, lives with his girl-friend, born in Iran, has lived in Britain for nineteen years.
6. Male takeaway employee, forty-two years old, cousin of 5, married to 19, lives with his wife and two children, born in Iran, has lived in Britain for five years.
7. Female restaurant owner, forty-six years old, married, lives with husband and two children, born in Iran, has lived in Britain for twenty-four years.
8. Male restaurant manager, twenty-three years old, son of 7, single, lives with his parents.
9. Male takeaway owner, forty-seven years old, divorced, lives alone, born in Iran, has lived in Britain for thirteen years.
10. Male takeaway owner, forty-three years old, single, lives alone, born in Iran, has lived in Britain for twelve years.
11. Male takeaway owner, thirty-two years old, married, lives with wife and one child, born in Iran, has lived in Britain for twenty years.
12. Female co-owner of takeaway, thirty-one years old, wife of 11, born in Britain, English parents.
13. Male takeaway owner, forty-two years old, married to 25, lives with wife and two children, born in Iran, has lived in Britain for eight years.
14. Female takeaway owner and part-time mature student, forty-eight years old, sister of 25, single, born in Iran, has lived in Britain for twelve years.

15. Male dental technician, thirty-one years old, single, lives alone, born in Iran, has lived in Britain for fifteen years

Domestic food-work, health and identity

16. Housewife, thirty-four years old, married to 2, born in Iran, has lived in Britain for ten years.
17. Housewife, sister of 2, forty-three years old, married, lives with husband and two children, born in Iran, has lived in Britain for seven years.
18, Housewife, thirty-two years old, married to 4, born in Iran, has lived in Britain for eleven years.
19. Housewife, forty years old, married to 6, born in Iran, has lived in Britain for five years.
20. Male university lecturer, forty-eight years old, married, lives with wife and three children, born in Iran, has lived in Britain for eighteen years.
21. Unemployed male, fifty-one years old, married, lives with wife and two children, born in Iran, has lived in Britain for sixteen years.
22. Female factory machinist, forty-eight years old, wife of 21, born in Iran, has lived in Britain for sixteen years.
23. Male postgraduate student, forty-two years old, married, lives with his wife and two children, born in Iran, has lived in Britain for four years.
24. Housewife and part-time word processor, thirty-eight years old, wife of 23, born in Iran, has lived in Britain for four years.
25. Housewife, thirty-nine years old, married to 13, born in Iran, has lived in Britain for eight years.
26, Female hairdresser, forty-five years old, divorced, lives with partner, born in Iran, came to Britain as a teenager.
27. Female postgraduate student, twenty-nine years old, married, lives with husband and two children, born in Iran, has lived in Britain for five years.
28. Male postgraduate student, thirty-one years old, husband of 27, born in Iran, has lived in Britain for five years.
29. Male postgraduate student, twenty-eight years old, married, lives with wife and one child, born in Iran, has lived in Britain for two years.
30. Housewife, twenty-seven years old, married to 29, born in Iran, has lived in Britain for two years.
31. Male postgraduate student, 30 years old, married, lives with wife and one child, born in Iran, has lived in Britain for 3 years
32. Housewife, twenty-seven years old, married to 31, born in Iran, has lived in Britain for three years.

Gender relations

2. Male takeaway owner, forty-two years old, married, lives with wife and one child, born in Iran, has lived in Britain for twenty years.

3. Male food wholesaler and entrepreneur, forty-five years old, married to 17, born in Iran, has lived in Britain for eight years.

4. Male takeaway owner, forty-one years old, married, lives with his wife and two children, born in Iran, has lived in Britain for twenty years.

5. Male takeaway owner, forty years old, single, lives with his girl-friend, born in Iran, has lived in Britain for nineteen years.

6. Male takeaway employee, forty-two years old, cousin of 5, married, lives with his wife and two children, born in Iran, has lived in Britain for five years

13. Male takeaway owner, forty-two years old, married to 25, lives with wife and two children, born in Iran, has lived in Britain for eight years.

14. Female takeaway owner and part-time mature student, 48 years old, sister of 25, single, born in Iran, has lived in Britain for twelve years.

16. Housewife, thirty-four years old, married to 2, born in Iran, has lived in Britain for ten years.

17. Housewife, sister of 2, forty-three years old, married, lives with husband and two children, born in Iran, has lived in Britain for seven years.

18. Housewife, thirty-two years old, married to 4, born in Iran, has lived in Britain for eleven years.

19. Housewife, forty years old, married to 6, born in Iran, has lived in Britain for five years.

21. Unemployed male, fifty-one years old, married, lives with wife and two children, born in Iran, has lived in Britain for sixteen years.

22. Female factory machinist, forty-eight years old, wife of 21, born in Iran, has lived in Britain for sixteen years.

25. Housewife, thirty-nine years old, married to 13, born in Iran, has lived in Britain for eight years.

26. Female hairdresser, forty-five years old, divorced, lives with partner, born in Iran, came to Britain as a teenager.

27. Female postgraduate student, twenty-nine years old, married, lives with husband and two children, born in Iran, has lived in Britain for five years.

31. Male postgraduate student, thirty years old, married, lives with wife and one child, born in Iran, has lived in Britain for three years.

32. Housewife, 27 years old, married to 31, born in Iran, has lived in Britain for 3 years.

Children, food and identities

33. Schoolgirl, five year old, daughter of 2 and 16, born in Britain.
34. Schoolboy, sixteen years old, son of 17 and 3, born in Iran, has lived in Britain for seven years.
35. Schoolgirl, ten years old, daughter of 17 and 3, sister of 34, born in Iran, has lived in Britain for seven years.
36. Schoolgirl, nine years old, eldest daughter of 4 and 18, born in Britain.
37. Schoolboy, eleven years old, eldest son of 6 and 19, born in Iran, has lived in Britain for five years.
38. Female university student, seventeen years old, single, lives in shared accommodation, born in Iran, has lived in Britain for fourteen years.
39. Schoolboy, fourteen years old, elder son of 23 and 24, born in Iran, has lived in Britain for four years.
40. Schoolboy, eight years old, younger son of 23 and 24 and brother of 39, born in Iran, has lived in Britain for four years.
41. Schoolgirl, sixteen years old, born in Iran, has lived in Britain for thirteen years.
42. Schoolgirl, ten years old, daughter of 13 and 25, born in Iran, has lived in Britain for eight years.
43. Schoolboy, six years old, son of 13 and 25 and brother of 42, born in Britain.

BIBLIOGRAPHY

Adair, G. *Myths and Memories*, London: Fontana, 1986.

Afshah, H. *Women in the Middle East: Perceptions, Realities and Struggles for Liberation*, London: Macmillan, 1993.

Amit-Talai, V and Wulff, H. (eds.) *Youth Cultures. A Cross Cultural Perspective*, London: Routledge, 1995.

Back, L. *New Ethnicities and Urban Cultures. Racisms and Multiculture in Young Lives*. Race and Representation 2, London: University College London, 1996.

Bagheri, A. 'Psychiatric Problems among Iranian Immigrants in Canada', *Canadian Journal of Psychiatry* 37 (1992): 7–11.

Bakhtin, M. *The Dialogic Imagination,* trans. by Emerson, C. and Hosquist, M, Austin, Texas: University of Texas Press, 1981.

Bauman, Z. *Thinking Sociologically*, Oxford: Blackwell, 1990.

Baxter, S. and Raw, G. 'Fast Food, Fettered Work: Chinese Women in the Ethnic Catering Industry', in Westwood, S. and Bhachu, P. (eds.) *Enterprising Women. Ethnicity, Economy, and Gender Relations,* London: Routledge, 1988.

Beardsworth, A. and Keil, T. *Sociology on the Menu: An Invitation to the Study of Food and Society,* London: Routledge, 1997.

Beck, L. and Keddie, N. (eds.) *Women in the Muslim World,* London: Harvard University Press, 1979.

Benson, S. *Ambiguous Ethnicity. Interracial Families in London,* Cambridge: Cambridge University Press, 1981.

Bhopal, R.S. 'Future Research on the Health of Ethnic Minorities: Back to Basics; a Personal View', *Ethnic Minorities Health,* 1, no. 3 (1989): i–iii.

Bhopal, R.S. 'The Health of Ethnic Minorities: Problems in Research, Policy-making and Health-care Planning', paper given to International Child Health Group University Hospital of Wales, Cardiff, 9 October 1992.

Blaxter, M. *Health and Lifestyles,* London: Tavistock/Routledge, 1990.

Boakes R.A., Popplewell D.A., and Burton M.J. *Food, Physiology and Learned Behaviour. Acquisition of Food Acceptance Patterns in Children,* Chichester: Wiley and Sons, 1987.

Booth, D.A., Conner, M.T. and Marie, S. 'Sweetness and Food Selection: Measurement of Sweeteners' Effects on Acceptance', in Dobbing, J. (ed.) *Sweetness,* Berlin: Springer-Verlag, 1987.

Bourdieu, P. *Distinction: A Social Critique of the Judgement of Taste,* London: Routledge, 1984.

Bradby H. 'Of heating and Heart Attacks: Understandings of Health and Food among Young British Asian Women'. Paper given to B.S.A. Medical Sociology Group, 22–24 September 1995, York.

Bradby, H. 'Health, Eating and Heart Attacks: Glaswegian Punjabi Women's Thinking about Everyday Food', in Caplan, P. (ed.) *Food, Health and Identity,* London: Routledge, 1997.

Brannen, J. and O'Brien, M. *Children in Families: Research and Policy.* London: Falmer Press, 1996.

Brannen, J., Dodd, K., Oakley, A. and Storey, P. *Young People, Health and Family Life,* Buckingham: Open University Press, 1994.

Brown, J. and Kerns, V. *In Her Prime. A New View of Middle-Aged Women,* Massachusetts: Bergin & Garvey Publishers, 1985.

Bryman, A. *Quantity and Quality in Social Research,* London: Unwin Hyman, 1988.

Bull, N.L. 'Dietary Habits of 15 to 25 Year Olds'. *Human Nutrition: Applied Nutrition,* 39A, Suppl. 1 (1985): 1–68.

Caglar, A. 'McKebap: Doner Kebap and Turkish Identity in Berlin'. Paper given at The Global and the Local Consumption and European Identity. Fourth Conference on Research in Consumption. Amsterdam, 8–11 September 1993.

Caines, R. (ed.) *Fast Food and Home Delivery Outlets, Keynote Reports, An Industry Sector Overview,* 11th Edn., London: Key Note Publications, 1994.

Caplan, P. (ed) *Food, Health and Identity,* London: Routledge, 1997.

Charles, N. and Kerr, M. 'Food for Feminist Thought', *Sociological Review* 34, no. 3 986): 537–72.

Charles N. and Kerr, M. *Women, Food and Families.* Manchester: Manchester University Press, 1988.

Clinton-Davis, L. and Fassil, Y. 'Health and Social Problems of Refugees', *Social Sciences* 35, no. 4 (1992): 507–13.

Colliver Rice, C. *Persian Women and their Ways.* London: Seeley, Service and Co, 1923.

Cornwall, A. and Lindisfarne, N. 'Dislocating Masculinity: Gender, Power and Anthropology', in Cornwall, A. and Lindisfarne, N. (eds.) *Dislocating Masculinity.* Comparative Ethnographies, London: Routledge, 1994.

Counihan, C.M. 'Female Identity, Food and Power in Contemporary Florence'. *Anthropological Quarterly* 61, no. 2 (1988): 51–62.

Cowan, J. 'Going out for Coffee? Contesting the Grounds of Gendered Pleasures in Everyday Sociability', Chapter 8 in Loizos, P. and Papataxiarchis, E. (eds.) *Contested Identities: Gender and Kinship in Modern Greece,* Princeton: Princeton University Press, 1991.

Coxon, T. 'Men in the Kitchen: Notes from a Cookery Class', in *The Sociology of food and Eating.* Murcott, A. (ed.). Aldershot: Gower, 1983.

Cruikshank, J.K. and Beevers, D. G. (eds.) *Ethnic Factors in Health and Disease,* London: Wright, 1989.

Csikzentmihalyi, M. and Rochberg-Halton, E. *The Meaning of Things,* Cambridge: Cambridge University Press, 1981.

Csordas, T.J. (ed.) *Embodiment and Experience: The Existential Ground of Culture and Self,* Cambridge: Cambridge University Press, 1994.

Davis, C.M. 'Results of the Self-selection of Diets by Young Children', *Canadian Medical Association Journal* 41 (1939): 257–61.

Davison, C., Smith, G.D. and Frankel, S. 'Lay Epidemiology and the Prevention Paradox: the Implications of Coronary Candidacy for Health Education', *Sociology of Health and Illness* 13, no. 1 (1991): 1–19.

De Groot, J. 'Gender, Discourse and Ideology in Iranian Studies: Towards a New Scholarship', in Kandiyoti, D. (ed.) *Gendering the Middle East. Emerging Perspectives,* New York: Syracuse University Press, 1996.

DeVault, M.L. *Feeding the Family: The Social Organisation of Caring as Gendered Work.* Chicago: Chicago University Press, 1991.

Dorman, W.A. 'Iranian People v. U.S. News Media: a Case of Libel', *Race and Class* 21, no. 1 (1979): 57–66.

Douglas, M. *Purity and Danger: An Analysis of Concepts of Pollution and Taboo,* London: Routledge and Kegan Paul, 1970.

Douglas. M. 'Food as a System of Communication', in Douglas. M. *In the Active Voice,* London: Routledge, 1982.

Driver, C. *The British at Table 1940–80,* London: Howarth Press, 1983.

Drewnowski, A. and Schwartz, M. 'Invisible Fats: Sensory Assessment of Sugar/fat Mixtures', *Appetite* 14 (1990): 203–17.

Dubos, R. 'Mirage of Health', in *Health and Disease. A Reader.*, Black, N., Boswell, D., Gray, A., Murphy, S. and Popay J. (eds.) Milton Keynes: Open University Press, 1992.

Ekstrom, M. 'Class and Gender in the Kitchen', in Fürst, E.L., Prattala, R., Ekstrom, M., Holm, L. and Kjaernes I. (eds.) *Palatable Worlds. Sociocultural Food Studies,* Oslo: Solum Forlag, 1991.

Epstein, A.L. *Ethos and Identity: Three studies in Ethnicity.* London: Tavistock Publications, 1978.

Esquivel, L. *Like Water for Chocolate,* London: Black Swan, 1993.

Falk, P. *The Consuming Body,* London: Sage, 1994.

Farb, P. and Amelagos, G. *Consuming Passions: The Anthropology of Eating,* Boston, Mass.: Houghton Mifflin, 1980.

Farman Farmaian, S. with Munker, D. *Daughter of Persia: A Woman's Journey from her Father's Harem through the Islamic Revolution,* London: Corgi, 1992.

Fathi, A. (ed.) *Iranian Refugees and Exiles Since Khomeini,* Calgary: Mazda Publishers, 1991.

Featherstone, M. 'The Body in Consumer Culture', in Featherstone, M., Hepworth, M. and Turner, B. (eds.) *The Body: Social Process and Cultural Theory.* London: Sage, 1991.

Fine, G.A. 'The Culture of Production: Aesthetic Choices and Constraints in Culinary Work', *American Journal of Sociology* 97, no. 5 (1992): 1268–94.

Finkelstein, J. *Dining Out: A Sociology of Modern Manners,* Cambridge: Polity Press, 1989.

Fischer, M.J. 'On Changing the Concept and Position of Persian Women', in Beck, L. and Keddie, N. (eds.) *Women in the Muslim World,* London: Harvard University Press, 1979.

Fischer, M.J. *Iran: From Religious Dispute to Revolution,* Harvard Studies in Cultural Anthropology, 3, Cambridge, Mass.: Harvard University Press, 1980.

Fischer, M.M.J. and Abedi, M. *Debating Muslims. Cultural Dialogues in Postmodernity and Tradition,* London: University of Winsconsin Press, 1990.

Fischler, C. 'Food Habits, Social Change and the Nature/culture Dilemma', *Social Science Information* 19, no. 6 (1980): 937–53.

Fischler, C. 'Food, Self and Identity', *Social Science Information* 27, no. 2 (1988): 275–92.

Fishlock, T. 'Hot Spots', *The Telegraph Magazine,* 23 July 1994.

Fragner, B. 'From the Caucasus to the Roof of the World: A Culinary Adventure', in Zubaida, S. and Tapper, R. (eds.) *Culinary Cultures of the Middle East,* London: I.B. Taurus, 1994a.

Fragner, B. 'Social Reality and Culinary Fiction: the Perspective of Cookbooks from Iran and Central Asia,in Zubaida, S. and Tapper, R. (eds.) *Culinary Cultures of the Middle East,* London: I.B. Taurus, 1994b.

Frankenberg, R. 'Sickness as Cultural Performance', *International Journal of Health Services* 16 (1986): 603–26.

Fuller, G.E. *The Centre of the Universe: The Geopolitics of Iran,* Oxford: Westview Press, 1991.

Fürst, E.L. 'Food, Identity and Gender. A Story of Ambiguity', in Fürst, E.L., Prattala, R., kstrom, M, Holm, L and Kjaernes (eds.) *Palatable Worlds. Sociocultural Food Studies,* Oslo: Solum Forlag, 1991.

Gardner, K. '*Desh-Bidesh*: Sylheti Images of Home and Away', *Man* 28, no. 1 (1993): 1–15.

Gardner, K. *Global Migrants Local Lives. Travel and Transformation in Rural Bangladesh,* Oxford Studies in Social and Cultural Anthropology, Oxford: Clarendon Press, 1995.

Gefou-Madianou, D. (ed.) *Alcohol, Gender and Culture,* London: Routledge, 1992.

Ghvamshahidi, Z. 'The Linkage between Iranian Patriarchy and the Informal Economy in Maintaining Women's Subordinate Roles in Home-based Carpet Production', *Women's Studies International Forum* 18, no. 2 (1995): 135–51.

Gilanshah, F. 'The Formation of Iranian Community in the Twin Cities from 1983–89', *Wisconsin Sociologist* 27, no. 4 (1990): 11–17.

Goffman, E. *Stigma. Notes on the Management of Spoiled Identity.,*Harmondsworth, Penguin, 1968.

Good, B.J. 'The Heart of What's the Matter: The Semantics of Illness in Iran', *Culture, Medicine and Psychiatry* 1 (1977): 25–58.

Greenwood, B. 'Cold or Spirits? Choice and Ambiguity in Morocco's Pluralist System', *Social Science and Medicine* 15B (1981): 219–35.

Grindulis, H., Scott, P.H., Belton, N.R. and Wharton, B.A. 'Combined deficiency of iron and vitamin D in Asian toddlers', *Archives of Disease in Childhood* 61 (1986): 843–48.

Guppy, S. *The Blindfold Horse. Memories of a Persian Childhood,* London: Minerva, 1992.

Hall, S. 'Cultural Identity and Diaspora', in Rutherford, J. (ed.) *Identity, Community, Culture, Difference,* London: Lawrence and Wishart, 1990.

Haraway, D. 'A Manifesto for Cyborgs: Science, Technology and Socialist Feminism in the 1980's', in Nicholson, L.J. (ed.) *Feminism/Postmoderism,* Thinking Gender Series, London: Routledge, 1990.

Haraway, D.J. *Simians, Cyborgs and Women:The Reinvention of Nature,* London: Routledge, 1991.

Harbottle, L. 'When Counselling becomes Spiritual Abuse', *Anglicans for Renewal Magazine* Spring (1993): 19–22.

Harbottle, L. 'Feminism and Medical Anthropology', *British Medical Anthropology Review* 2, no. 2 (1994): 28–40.

Harbottle, L. *'Palship', Parties and Pilgrimage: Kinship, Community Formation and Self-Transformation of Iranian Migrants to Britain. Working Paper No. 9: Representations of Places and Identities,* Keele: Keele University Press, 1995.

Harbottle, L. Towards a Culturally Sensitive Research Approach. *Scandinavian Journal of Nutrition* 40, no. 2, Suppl 31 (1996): S125–26.

Harbottle, L. 'Beyond Cultural Sensitivity: Employing Ethnographic Techniques to Improve the Effectiveness and Outcomes of Community Nutrition Surveys', in Kohler, B.M., Feichtinger, E., Dowler, E. and Winkler, G. (eds.) *Public Health and Nutrition,* Berlin: Ed. Sigma (1999).

Harbottle, L. and Duggan, M.B. 'Comparative Study of the Dietary Characteristics of Asian Toddlers with Iron Deficiency in Sheffield', *Journal of Human Nutrition and Dietetics* 5 (1992): 501–12.

Harris, M. *Good to Eat: Riddles of Food and Culture,* London: Allen and Unwin, 1986.

Harris, R.J., Armstrong, D., Ali, R. and Loynes, A. 'Nutritional Survey of Bangladeshi Children Aged under 5 Years in the London Borough of Tower Hamlets', *Archives of Disease in Childhood* 58 (1983): 428–32.

Hoffman, D.M. 'Beyond Conflict: Culture, Self and Intercultural Learning Among Iranians in the U.S.', *International Journal of Intercultural Relations* 14, no. 3 (1990), 275–99.

Hoodfar, H. 'The Veil in Their Minds and on Our Heads: The Persistence of Colonial Images of Muslim Women', *Resources for Feminist Research* 22, no. 3/4 (1993): 5–18.

James, A. 'Confections, Concoctions and Conceptions', *Journal of the Anthropological Society* 10, no. 2 (1979): 83–95.

James, A. 'The Good, the Bad and the Delicious: the Role of Confectionery in British Society', *Sociological Review* 38, no. 4 (1990): 666–89.

James, A. 'How British is British Food? A View from Anthropology', in Caplan, P. (ed.) *Food, Health and Identity,* London: Routledge, 1997.

James, A. and Prout, A. *Constructing and Reconstructing Childhood. Contemporary Issues in the Sociological Study of Childhood,* London: Falmer Press, 1990.

Jamzadeh, L. and Mills, M. 'Iranian *Sofreh*: From Collective to Female Ritual', in Bynum, C.W., Harrell, S. and Richman, P. (eds.) *Gender and Religion: On the Complexity of Symbols,* Boston: Beacon Press, 1986.

Jansson, S. 'Food Practices and Division of Domestic Labour. A Comparison between British and Swedish Households', *Sociological Review* 43, no. 3 (1995): 462–77.

Jenks, C. *Culture: Key Ideas,* London: Routledge, 1993.

Jenkins, R. *Social Identity: Key Ideas,* London: Routledge, 1996.

Johnston, J.P. *A Hundred Years Eating. Food, Drink and the Daily Diet in Britain Since t the Late Nineteenth Century,* Dublin: Gill and Macmillan, 1977.

Kalka, I. 'The Changing Food Habits of Gujaratis in Britain', *Journal of Human Nutrition and Dietetics* 1 (1988): 329–35.

Kallarackal, A.M. and Herbert, M. 'The Happiness of Indian Migrant Children', *New Society* 35, no. 699 (1976): 422–23.

Kamalkhani, Z. *Iranian Immigrants and Refugees in Norway, Bergen Studies in Social Anthropology, No. 43,* Bergen: University of Bergen, 1988.

Kamalkhani, Z. 'Iranians in Norway: Adaptation and Community Formation', *Migration World Magazine,* 19, no. 2 (1991): 8–12.

Kandel, R.F and Pelto, G.H. 'The Health Food Movement', in *Nutritional Anthropology: Contemporary Approaches to Diet and Culture,* New York: Redgrave Publishing Company, 1980.

Kandiyoti, D. *Gendering the Middle East. Emerging Perspectives,* New York: Syracuse University Press, 1996.

Kerr, M. and Charles, N. 'Servers and Providers: The Distribution of Food within a Family', *Sociological Review* 34, no. 1 (1986): 115–55.

Khare, R.S. 'Food as Nutrition and Culture: Notes Towards an Anthropological Methodology', *Social Science Information* 19, no. 3 (1980): 519–42.

Kupers, T.A. *Revisioning Men's Lives,* New York: The Guildford Press, 1993.

Lalonde, M.P. 'Deciphering a Meal Again, or the Anthropology of Taste', *Social Science Information* 31, no. 1(1992): 69–86.

Lask, B. and Bryant-Waugh, R. (eds.) *Childhood Onset Anorexia Nervosa and Related Eating Disorders,* Hove: Lawrence Erlbaum, 1993.

Law, J. 'How Much of Society Can the Sociologist Digest at One Sitting? The "Macro" and the "Micro" Revisited for the Case of Fast Food', *Studies in Symbolic Interaction* 5 (1984): 171–96.

Leach, E. 'Anthropological Aspects of Language: Animal Categories and Verbal Abuse', in Lennenberg, E.H. (ed.) *New Directions in the Study of Language,* Cambridge, Mass.: MIT Press, 1964.

Leach, R. (1998) *Consumption and Embodiment, Salford University Working Papers, Series 8,* Salford, Salford University Press.

Leichty, M. 'Media, Markets and Modernisation. Youth Identities and the Experience of Modernity in Kathmandu, Nepal', in Amit-Talai, V. and Wulff, H. (eds.) *outh Cultures. A Cross Cultural Perspective,* London: Routledge, 1995.

Leidner, R. *Fast Food, Fast Talk,* California: University of California Press, 1993.

Lévi-Strauss, C. 'The Culinary Triangle', *New Society* 22 (1966): 937–41.

Lévi-Strauss, C. *Structural Anthropology*, vol 1, Harmondsworth: Allen Lane, Penguin Press, 1968.

Light, I., Sabagh, G., Bozorgmehr, M.and Der-Martirosian, C. 'Internal Ethnicity in the Ethnic Economy', *Ethnic and Racial Studies* 16, no. 4 (1993): 581–97.

Light, I., Sabagh, G., Bozorgmehr, M. and Der-Martirosian, C. 'Beyond the Ethnic Enclave Economy', *Social Problems* 41, no. 1 (1994): 65–80.

Lipson, J.G. 'The Health and Adjustment of Iranian Immigrants', *Western Journal of Nursing Research* 14, no. 1 (1992): 10–29.

Lock, M. *East Asian Medicine in Urban Japan. Comparative Studies of Health Systems and Medical Care. Number 4*, Berkeley: University of California Press, 1980.

Lupton, D. *Food, the Body and the Self*, London: Sage, 1996.

Malinowski, B. *Coral Gardens and their Magic*, New York: American Book Company, 1935.

Mares, P., Henly, A. and Baxter, C. *Health Care in Multiracial Britain*, Cambridge: Health Education Council/National Extension College, 1985.

Margold, J.A. 'Narratives of Masculinity and Transnational Migration: Filipino Workers in the Middle East', in Ong, A. and Peletz, M.G. (eds.) *Bewitching Women, Pious Men. Gender and Body Politics in Southeast Asia*, Berkeley: University of California Press, 1995.

Mars, V. 'Spaghetti - but not on Toast! Italian food in London', in Mars A. and Mars V. *Food in Motion. The Migration of Foodstuffs and Cookery Techniques, The Oxford Symposium Volume 1*, Totnes: Prospect Books, 1993.

Mauss, M. *The Gift: The Form and Reason for Exchange in Archaic Societies*, London: Routledge, 1950.

McElinney, B. 'An Economy of Affect: Objectivity, Masculinity and the Gendering of Police Work', in Cornwall, A. and Lindisfarne, N. (eds.) *Dislocating Masculinity. Comparative Ethnographies*, London: Routledge, 1994.

Mead M. 'Dietary Patterns and food habits', *Journal Of the American Dietetic Association* 19 (1943): 1–5.

Medical Research Council *Annual Report*, Glasgow, Medical Research Council, 1996.

Mennell, S. *All Manners of Food: Eating and Taste in England and France from the Middle Ages to the Present*, Oxford: Blackwell, 1985.

Mennell, S., Murcott, A., and Van Otterloo, A.H. *The Sociology of Food: Eating, Diet d Culture*, London: Sage, 1992.

Merleau-Ponty, M. *Phenomenology of Perception*, London: Routledge and Kegan- Paul, 1962.

Messer, E. 'Hot-cold Classification: Theoretical and Practical Implications of a Mexican Study', *Social Science and Medicine* 15B (1981): 133–45.

Messner, M.A. and Sabo, D.F. *Sport, Men and the Gender Order. Critical Feminist Perspectives*, Champaign, Illinois: Human Kinetic Books, 1990.

Miller, S. (ed.) *Ethnic Foods: U.K. Catering Market, Industry Trends and Forecasts, Keynote Market Review*, 2nd edn., London: Key Note Publications, 1986.

Miller, S. (ed.) *Restaurants: U.K. Catering Market, Industry Trends and Forecasts, Keynote Market Review,* 7th edn., London: Key Note Publications, 1994.

Mintz, S. *Sweetness and Power: the Place of Sugar in Modern History,* New York: Viking Press, 1985.

Moore. H. *A Passion for Difference. Essays in Anthropology and Gender,* Cambridge: Polity Press, 1994.

Murcott, A. 'On the social significance of the "Cooked Dinner" in South Wales', *Social Science Information* 21, no. 4/5 (1982): 677–96

Murcott, A. *The Sociology of Food and Eating: Essays on the Social Significance of Food,* Aldershot: Gower, 1983.

Murcott, A. 'Sociological and Social Anthropological Approaches to Food and Eating', *World Review of Nutrition and Dietetics* 55 (1988): 1–40.

Murcott, A. 'Family Meals: A Thing of the Past?' in Caplan, P. (ed.) *Food, Health and Identity,* London: Routledge, 1997.

Murphy, R. *The Body Silent,* New York: Henry Holt and Co, 1987.

O'Laughlin, B. 'Mediation of Contradiction: Why Mbum Women Do Not Eat Chicken', in Rosaldo, M. and Lamphere, L. (eds.) *Woman, Culture and Society,* Stanford: Stanford University Press, 1974.

Oakley, A. *Becoming a Mother,* Oxford: Martin Robertson, 1979.

Office of Population and Census Statistics *1991 Census, Great Britain Monitor,* O.P.C.S. Series CEN91 NR1, London: H.M.S.O, 1993.

Okely, J. *The Traveller Gypsies,* Cambridge, Cambridge University Press, 1983.

Ong, A. and Peletz, M.G. *Bewitching Women, Pious Men. Gender and Body Politics in Southeast Asia,* Berkeley: University of California Press, 1995.

Ortner, S.B. 'Is Female to Male as Nature is to Culture?' in Rosaldo, M. and Lamphere, L. (eds.) *Woman, Culture & Society,* Stanford; Stanford University Press, 1974.

Ortner, S.B. and Whitehead, H. (eds.) *Sexual Meanings. The Cultural Construction of Gender and Sexuality,* Cambridge: Cambridge University Press, 1989.

Pacey, P.J. 'Nutritional Patterns and Deficiencies, in Cruikshank, J.K. and Beevers, D. G. (eds.) *Ethnic Factors in Health and Disease,* London: Wright, 1989.

Parker, D. 'Encounters Across the Counter: Young Chinese People in Britain', *New Community* 20, no. 4 (1994): 621–34.

Payne, M. and Payne, B. *Eating out in the U.K.: Market Structure, Consumer Attitudes and Prospects for the 1990s,* Economist Intelligence Unit, Special Report No. 2169, London: Economist Intelligence Unit Ltd, 1993.

Pearson, M. 'Racist Notions of Ethnicity and Culture in Health Education', in Rodmell, S. and Watt, A. (eds.) *The Politics of Health Education: Raising the Issues,* London: Routledge, 1986.

Pearson, M. 'Sociology of Race and Health', in Cruikshank, J.K. and Beevers, D.G. (eds.) *Ethnic Factors in Health and Disease,* London: Wright, 1989.

Peletz, M.G. 'Neither Reasonable Nor Responsible: Contrasting Representations of Masculinity in a Malay Society', in Ong, A. and Peletz, M.G.

(eds.) *Bewitching Women, Pious Men. Gender and Body Politics in Southeast Asia*, Berkeley: University of California Press, 1995.

Pliskin, K. *Silent Boundaries. Cultural Constraints on Sickness and Diagnosis of Iranians in Israel.* New Haven: Yale University Press, 1987.

Pong, N.N. 'An Empirical Study of Attitudes towards a Chinese Restaurant in Sheffield' (MSc Diss., Sheffield University), 1986

Radcliffe-Brown, A.R. *The Andaman Islanders*, Cambridge: Cambridge University Press, 1922.

Ramzani, R.K. *Revolutionary Iran, Challenge and Response in the Middle East*, Baltimore: John Hopkins University Press, 1986.

Rassam, A. 'Towards a Theoretical Framework For the Study of Women in the Arab World', in *Social Science Research and Women in the Arab World*, London: Pinter, 1984.

Reed-Danahay, D. 'Champagne and Chocolate: Taste and Inversion in a French Wedding Ritual', *American Anthropologist* 98, no. 4 (1996): 750–61.

Richards, A.J. *Land, Labour and Diet in Northern Rhodesia*, London: Oxford University Press, 1939.

Richardson, A. and Bowden, J. *A New Dictionary of Christian Theology*, London: S.C.M. Press, 1983.

Roosens, E.E. *Creating Ethnicity: The Process of Ethnogenesis*, Frontiers of Anthropology, Vol. 5, London: Sage, 1989.

Rosaldo, M.Z. 'Woman, Culture and Society: a Theoretical Overview', In Rosaldo, M.Z. and Lamphere, L. (eds.) *Woman, Culture and Society*, Stanford: Stanford University Press, 1974.

Rosaldo, M.Z. 'The Use and Abuse of Anthropology: Reflections on Feminism and Cross-cultural Understanding', *Signs: Journal of Women in Culture and Society* 5, no. 3 (1980): 389–417.

Rozin, P. 'The Use of Characteristic Flavourings in Human Culinary practice', in Apt, C.M. (ed.) *Flavour: Its Chemical, Behavioural and Commercial Aspects*, Boulder, CO: Westview Press, 1978.

Rozin, P. 'Human Food Selection: The Interaction of Biology, Culture, and Individual Experience', in Barker, L.M. (ed.) *The Psychobiology of Human Food Selection*, Chichester: Ellis Horwood, 1982.

Rozin, P., 'Sweetness, Sensuality, Sin, Safety and Socialisation: Some Speculations', in Dobbing, J. (ed.) *Sweetness*, Berlin: Springer-Verlag, 1987.

Rozin, P. 'The Role of Learning in the Acquisition of Food Preferences by Humans', in Shepherd, R. (ed.) *Handbook of the Psychophysiology of Human Eating*, Chichester: Wiley, 1989.

Rozin, P., Pelchat, M.L. and Fallon, A.E. 'Psychological Factors Influencing Food Choice', in Ritson, C., Gofton, L. and McKenzie J. (eds.) *The Food Consumer*, London: Wiley and Sons, 1986.

Rutherford, J. 'A Place Called Home: Identity and the Cultural Politics of Difference', in Rutherford, J (ed.) *Identity. Community, Culture, Difference.* London: Lawrence and Wishart, 1990.

Sansone. L. 'The Making of a Black Youth Culture. Lower Class Young Men of Surinamese Origin in Amsterdam', in Amit-Talai, V. and Wulff,

H. (eds.) *Youth Cultures. A Cross Cultural Perspective,* London: Routledge, 1995.

Scheper-Hughes, N. *Death Without Weeping: The Violence of Everyday Life in Brazil,* London: University of California Press, 1993.

Scott, T.R. and Giza, B.K. 'Neurophysiological Aspects of Sweetness,' in Dobbing, J. (ed.) *Sweetness,* Berlin: Springer-Verlag, 1987.

Sered, S.S. 'Food and Holiness: Cooking as a Sacred Act among Middle-Eastern Jewish Women', *Anthropological Quarterly* 61, no. 3 (1988): 129–39.

Shaida, M. *The Legendary Cuisine of Persia,* Henley on Thames: Lieuse Books, 1992.

Shelton, A. 'A Theatre for Eating, Looking and Thinking: The Restaurant as Symbolic Space', *Sociological Spectrum* 10, no. 4 (1990): 507–26.

Shilling, C. *The Body and Social Theory,* London: Sage, 1993.

Sparrow, K.H. and Chretien, D.M. 'The Social Distance Perceptions of Racial and Ethnic Groups by College Students: A Research Note', *Sociological Spectrum* 13 (1993): 277–88.

Sreberny-Mohammadi, A. and Mohammadi, A. *Small Media, Big Revolution. Communication, Culture and the Iranian Revolution.* London: University of Minnesota Press, 1994

Strathern, M. *Partial Connections,* Savage, Maryland: Rowman and Littlefield, 1991.

Synott, A. *The Body Social: Symbolism, Self and Society.* London: Routledge, 1993.

Tan, S.P. and Wheeler, E. 'Concepts Relating to Health and Food Held by Chinese Women in London, *Ecology of Food and Nutrition* 13 (1983): 37–49.

Tapper, R. and Tapper, N. '"Eat This, It'll Do You a Power of Good": Food and Commensality among Durrani Pashtuns', *American Ethnologist* 13 no. 1 (1986): 62–79.

Tapper, R. 'Ethnic Identities and Social Categories in Iran and Afghanistan', in Tonkin, E., McDonald, M. and Chapman, M. (eds.) *History and Ethnicity, A.S.A. Monographs, No. 27.* London: Routledge, 1989.

Tapper, R. and Zubaida, S. 'Introduction' to Zubaida, S. and Tapper, R. (eds.) *Culinary Cultures of the Middle East,* London: I.B. Taurus, 1994.

Theophano, K. and Curtis, K. 'Sisters, Mothers and Daughters: Food Exchange and Reciprocity in an Italian-American Community', in Sharman, A., Theophano, K., Curtis, K. and Messer, E. (eds.) *Diet and Domestic Life in Society,* Philadelphia: Temple University Press, 1991.

Torab, A. 'Piety as Gendered Agency: A Study of *Jalaseh* Ritual Discourse in an Urban Neighbourhood in Iran', *The Journal of the Royal Anthropological Association* 2, no. 2 (1996): 235–52.

Turner, V. *From Ritual to Theatre,* New York: P.A.J. Publications, 1982.

Twigg, J. 'Vegetarianism and the Meanings of Meat', in Murcott, A. (ed.) *The Sociology of Food and Eating,* Aldershot: Gower, 1983.

Tze Ching, L. 'Ethnic Enterprise in the Kansas City Metropolitan Area: The Chinese', (PhD Diss., University of Kansas), 1990.

Walton, J.K. *Fish and Chips and the British Working Class, 1870–1940,* Leicester: Leicester University Press, 1992.

Warde, A. 'Changing Vocabularies of Taste, 1967–92: Discourses about Food Preparation', *British Food Journal* 96, no. 9 (1994): 22–25.

Warde, A. 'Afterword: The Future of the Sociology of Consumption' in Edgell, S., Hetherington, K. and Warde A. (eds.) *Consumption Matters,* Oxford: Blackwell, 1996.

Warde, A. *Consumption, Food and Taste: Culinary Antinomies and Commodity Culture,* London: Sage, 1997.

Warde, A. and Hetherington, K. 'English Households and Routine Food Practices', *Sociological Review* 42, no. 4 (1994): 758–78.

Warrington, S. and Storey, D.M. 'Comparative Studies of Asian and Caucasian Children, 2: Nutrition, Feeding Practices and Health', *European Journal of Clinical Nutrition* 42 (1988): 69–80.

Watson, J.L. 'The Chinese: Hong Kong Villagers in the British Catering Trade', in Watson, J.L. (ed.) *Between Two Cultures,* Oxford: Basil Blackwell, 1977.

Werbner, P. *The Migration Process: Capital, Gifts and Offerings among British Pakistanis,* Oxford: Berg, 1990a.

Werbner, P. 'Renewing an Industrial Past: British Pakistani Enterprises in Manchester. *Migration* 8 (1990b): 7–41.

Werbner, P. 'Essentialising Essentialism, Essentialising Silence. Ethnicity and Racism in Britain', in Wicker, H., Alber, J., Bolzman, C., Fibbi, R., Imhof, K. and Wimmer, A. (eds) *Migration, Ethnicity and State,* Zurich: Seismo, 1996.

Werbner, P. 'Introduction: The Dialectics of Cultural Hybridity', in Werbner, P. and Modood, T. (eds.) *Debating Cultural Hybridity. Multi-Cultural Identities and t he Politics of Anti-Racism,* London: Zed Books, 1997.

World Health Organisation *Plan of Action Implementing the Global Strategy for All.* Geneva, W.H.O., 1982.

Yates, P. 'Interpreting Life Texts and Negotiating Life Courses: Youth, Ethnicity and Culture', in Spencer, P. (ed.) *Anthropology and the Riddle of the Sphinx. Paradoxes of Change in the Life-course. A.S.A. Monographs 28,* London: Routledge, 1990.

Yudkin, J. *Sweet and Dangerous,* London: Bantam Books, 1972.

Zonis, M. *Majestic Failure: The Fall of the Shah,* Chicago: University of Chicago Press, 1991.

Zubaida, S. 'National, Communal and Global Dimensions in Middle Eastern Food Cultures', in Zubaida, S. and Tapper, R. (eds.) *Culinary Cultures of the Middle East,* London: I.B. Taurus, 1994a.

Zubaida, S. 'Rice in the Culinary Cultures of the Middle East', in Zubaida, S. and Tapper, R. (eds.) *Culinary Cultures of the Middle East,* London: I.B. Tauris, 1994b.

INDEX